An Atlas of
OBESITY AND
WEIGHT CONTROL

THE ENCYCLOPEDIA OF VISUAL MEDICINE SERIES

An Atlas of
OBESITY AND
WEIGHT CONTROL

George A. Bray, MD

Pennington Center
Baton Rouge, LA

The Parthenon Publishing Group
International Publishers in Medicine, Science & Technology

A CRC PRESS COMPANY
BOCA RATON   LONDON   NEW YORK   WASHINGTON, D.C.

Published in the USA by
The Parthenon Publishing Group
345 Park Avenue South, 10th Floor
New York, NY 10010, USA

Published in the UK and Europe by
The Parthenon Publishing Group
23–25 Blades Court
Deodar Road
London SW15 2NU, UK

Library of Congress Cataloging-in-Publication Data
An atlas of obesity and weight control/George A. Bray
    p. ; cm.-- (The encyclopedia of visual medicine series)
   Includes bibliographical references and index.
   ISBN 1-84214-049-3 (alk. paper)
    1. Obesity--Atlases. I. Title. II. Series
   [DNLM: 1. Obesity--etiology--Atlases. 2. Obesity--therapy--Atlases. 3. Obesity--prevention &
control--Atlases. 4. Weight Loss--Atlases. WD 210 B827 a 2002]
RC628 B6525 2002
616.3'98--dc21

British Library Cataloguing in Publication Data
An atlas of obesity and weight control.-(The encyclopedia of visual medicine series)
1. Obesity 2. Obesity-Treatment 3. Weight loss
I. Title
616.8'491

ISBN 1842140493

Typeset by Siva Math Setters, Chennai, India
Printed and bound by T. G. Hostench S. A., Spain

Contents

Foreword   7

Preface   9

Section I   A Review of Obesity   11

1   Realities in the treatment of obesity   13

2   Etiology of obesity   15
Energy balance and the controlled system
Afferent signals
The central controller
Efferent signals

3   Treatment of obesity   21
Historical perspective
Mechanisms of action
Currently available drugs
Side-effects
Features of an ideal drug

Section II   Obesity Illustrated   29

Index   131

Foreword

This book comes at a remarkably appropriate time as the World Health Organization not only highlights excess weight gain and obesity as the biggest unrecognized public health problem for mankind, but also now specifies it as one of the top dozen risk factors for the total health burden of the world.

Doctors have yet to take the extraordinary impact of obesity into their clinical practice, so it is particularly helpful to have at hand this invaluable compilation of data on the health consequences of obesity, its diverse pattern globally and how best to recognize the variety of genetic syndromes linked to obesity.

We are also now entering a new age in obesity management with a host of recent studies beautifully summarized in this book. They re-emphasize the benefits of sustained management of this condition. The specification of practical clinical care and how to track patients' responses with an emphasis on how to maximize the benefits of treatment are all encompassed in this beautifully produced atlas.

George Bray is the tireless world leader of obesity research and treatment, so it is a privilege to have this discerning summary of such a welter of data and new concepts. All clinicians would benefit from incorporating this new knowledge into their everyday practice.

W. Philip T. James
Chairman, International Obesity TaskForce
London, UK
November 2002

Preface

Obesity is a worldwide epidemic. It is also a disease. The cause is an imbalance between the energy we eat as food and the energy we need to keep our bodies running. This disease almost surely represents a change in the environment for which our ancient genes are not adapted. The pathology of obesity occurs at the level of the enlarged fat cell that we now know secretes many factors that can be harmful to other organs. This Atlas of Obesity and Weight Control is timely because it brings together in one place many of the lessons that I have tried to teach to those interested in this problem. It updates the epidemiological data and focuses on the mechanisms that may underlie the genetic and environmental factors that lead to this epidemic. Prevention is obviously the first line of defense against a disease so environmental in origin. The pictures in this book focus on a clinical approach to the problem when prevention fails.

The preparation of this book has stimulated me to bring together the best images I could find. It has had the careful editorial work of Ms Fiona Nitsche at Parthenon Publishing to whom I am grateful. It has also taken time away from family commitments, and I want to thank my wife, Marilyn, for her love and support. The valued contributions of many long-time collaborators were also important, and I want to thank Dr. David York, Dr. Frank Greenway, Dr. Donna Ryan, Dr. Barbara Hansen and Dr. Claude Bouchard. They can take much of the credit for this book, I will take the blame for any of the errors.

George A. Bray, MD
October 2002

Section 1 A Review of Obesity

1

Realities in the treatment of obesity

- Obesity is a chronic stigmatized disease that is increasing in prevalence

- Treatments rarely cure obesity

- The therapeutic armamentarium of physicians is limited and labors under the negative halo of amphetamine and treatment mishaps

- Drugs do not work when they are not taken

- Weight loss plateaus on any treatment when compensatory mechanisms come into play

- Frustration with plateaued weight loss that often averages less than 10% leads to discontinuation of therapy, weight regain, and attribution of failure to the weight loss program

Framing a treatment program in the field of obesity is best performed in the context of the realities that surround this disease. The first of these realities is that obesity is a chronic stigmatized disease that is increasing in prevalence. Both the World Health Organization and the National Heart, Lung and Blood Institute of the National Institutes of Health have labeled obesity an epidemic. More than 25% of adult Americans are now obese and the prevalence of obesity in children and adults has increased nearly 50% in the past decade. This epidemic is a time bomb for future development of diabetes and its many complications. As such, it deserves efforts for its prevention and, where needed, treatment. Given the size of the problem, there is an enormous opportunity for prevention and treatment.

As a disease, obesity has its pathology rooted in the enlargement of fat cells. The secretory products of these large fat cells produce most of the pathogenetic changes that result in the complications associated with obesity. Physicians and the health-care system have two strategies to deal with this problem.

The first is to prevent the development of obesity, or to treat it before the complications develop. Alternatively, the healthcare system can wait until the complications develop and then institute appropriate therapy. With the current high-quality therapies available to treat hypertension, diabetes mellitus and hypercholesterolemia, many physicians would prefer this latter strategy. However, if treatment for obesity were effective, the former approach would clearly be preferable. In one long-term trial, the incidence of new cases of diabetes was reduced to zero over 2 years in patients who lost and maintained a weight loss of 12% or more compared to an incidence of 8.5% for new cases of diabetes in those who did not lose weight. Thus, effective treatment can have a major impact in reducing the risk of developing serious diseases in the future.

One reason why most physicians are reluctant to treat obese patients is that their armamentarium is limited in the number of available compounds and in the effectiveness of this armamentarium. At the time of writing, there are only two agents approved for long-term use by the US Food and Drug Administration (FDA) and the European Committee on Proprietary Medicinal Products (CPMP). As monotherapy, either agent can produce a weight loss of 8–10%. However, to achieve the reduction in the rate of new cases of diabetes noted above, the weight loss needs to exceed 12%, a goal that cannot be achieved consistently with current monotherapy. Thus, there is a great need for new agents.

Obesity is a stigmatized disease. The common view is that obese people are lazy and weak-willed. If fat people just had willpower, they would push themselves away from the table and not be obese. This widely held view is shared by the public and by health professionals alike. This opinion of the obese is why many women clamour to be lean and well proportioned. The declining relative weight of centerfold models in Playboy and of women who are winners of the Miss America contest supports this view. It is a hurdle with which any new agent has to deal. Many physicians do not like to see obese patients come into their offices. Dealing with this problem poses a major challenge for governments and the health profession.

Two other issues aggravate the problem of treating obesity. The first is the 'negative halo' that surrounds the use of appetite suppressant drugs because amphetamine is addictive. Several drugs, including mazindol and dexfenfluramine for which there was never any evidence of drug abuse, were nonetheless restricted by the US Drug Enforcement Agency (DEA) because they had some chemical similarities on paper to amphetamine.

The second issue is the public concern about the plateau effect, which is reached when homeostatic mechanisms come into play. The therapeutic effect is reflected in a stable but lower body weight, without further change. There is an analogy with the treatment of hypertension. When an antihypertensive drug produces a decrease in blood pressure, there is a plateau at a new lower level. The antihypertensive drug has not lost its effect when the plateau occurs, but its effect is being counteracted by physiological mechanisms. In the treatment of obesity, a similar plateau in body weight is often viewed as a therapeutic failure of the weight loss treatment program. This is particularly so when weight is regained after treatment is stopped. These attitudes and biases need to change before any effective new therapy will become widely accepted.

The final issue concerns the disasters that recently befell many patients who took the combination of fenfluramine and phentermine. The aortic regurgitant lesions that occurred in up to 25% of the patients treated with this combination of drugs led many physicians to say 'I told you so' and 'I'm certainly glad I didn't use those drugs'. Much of this hostility will subside with time, but there will remain a residue of concern among some physicians, among regulators and among the public.

Where does the future lie? The epidemic of obesity is worldwide. If not curtailed it will be followed by an explosion of diabetes. Although there is a genetic basis for both obesity and diabetes, the current epidemic reflects the failure of our ancient genes to cope with our modern 'toxic' environment. To put it another way, our genes load the gun, the environment pulls the trigger.

Before effective action can be taken to overcome the epidemic of obesity two things need to happen. First, the public and the many governmental and non-governmental organizations need to become more focused on the implications of obesity and to organize effective strategies into national campaigns. Second, public attitudes toward overweight individuals need to shift from one of 'blame' for a weakness of character, to a recognition of the problem as a disease with significant associated risks.

2

Etiology of obesity

- Obesity is due to imbalance between energy intake and expenditure

- A feedback model can be used to understand the causes of energy imbalance

- Genetic causes of obesity in animals have human counterparts

Research over the past two decades has provided an unprecedented expansion of our knowledge about the physiological and molecular mechanisms regulating body fat. Perhaps the greatest impact has resulted from the cloning of genes corresponding to the five mouse monogenic obesity syndromes and the subsequent characterization of the pathways identified by these genetic entry points. Three of these genes (*ob*, *db* and *Ay*) have already led to potential drugs or drug targets currently in pharmaceutical development: leptin, leptin receptor, and the melanocortin-4 receptor (MC4R). In addition, extensive molecular and reverse genetic studies (mouse knockouts) have helped to establish other critical factors in energy balance, as well as validated or refuted the importance of previously identified pathways. This new information, combined with the increased recognition of obesity as a serious disease, has provided fuel to drug development for obesity across nearly the entire pharmaceutical industry. Potential strategies and specific targets for anti-obesity drugs that have resulted from these mechanistic insights are discussed below. As a framework for this discussion, I will use a feedback model. In such a system, there are afferent signals that inform central controls in the brain about the state of the external and internal environments related to food. In turn, this central controller transduces these messages into efferent control signals governing

the search for and acquisition of food, as well as modulating its subsequent disposal once inside the body. Finally, there is a control system that ingests, digests, absorbs, transports, stores, metabolizes and excretes the waste from the ingested food stuffs. In the drug discovery setting, each of these areas can be targeted. I will begin with the controlled system.

ENERGY BALANCE AND THE CONTROLLED SYSTEM

- Energy expenditure is related to fat free mass

- High carbohydrate oxidation predicts weight gain

- Fat, carbohydrate and protein can be separately regulated

- Low sympathetic activity is related to fatness

- β_3-Agonists are thermogenic drugs

- Uncoupling proteins mediate the response to β_3-agonists

- Peroxisome proliferator-activated receptor-γ (PPAR-γ) activation is one control for fat cell differentiation

The first Law of Thermodynamics tell us that obesity results from an imbalance between energy expenditure and energy intake. Energy expenditure can be divided into three major components. The largest of these is the 'resting' energy expenditure, followed quantitatively by physical activity and the thermic effect of food. Energy expenditure is most strongly associated with fat free body mass. A low rate of basal energy expenditure predicts future weight gain in some studies. The metabolic mixture oxidized by the body is related to the types of foods eaten, to the adaptive capacity of the body and to the rate of energy expenditure. To maintain energy balance requires that the mix of fuels eaten be oxidized. The capacity for storage of carbohydrate as glycogen is very limited and the capacity to store protein is also restricted. Only the fat stores can readily expand to accommodate increasing levels of energy intake above those required for daily energy needs. Several studies now show that a high rate of carbohydrate oxidation predicts future weight gain or regain after weight loss. One explanation for this is that, when carbohydrate oxidation is higher than the intake of carbohydrate, the body needs carbohydrate to replace the limited stores because it cannot convert fatty acids to carbohydrate and the conversion of amino acids to carbohydrate equivalents mobilizes protein stores. Obese individuals who have lost weight are less effective in increasing fat oxidation in the presence of a high fat diet than normal-weight individuals. Thus, dealing with control of fat oxidation and total oxidation may be one approach to obesity.

The energy expended in physical activity is directly related to body weight. Physical activity gradually declines with age, and maintaining a regular exercise program is difficult for many people, particularly as they get older. Adaptation to a change from a low to a higher fat diet takes time and can be accelerated by increasing exercise.

The thermic effect of food is the third component of energy expenditure. After ingesting food, there is a rise in energy expenditure which is about 10% of the day's energy expenditure. The sympathetic nervous system controls part of this process. The control of sympathetic activity and its noradrenergic output offers a possible strategy for treating obesity by raising energy expenditure. The thermic effect of food is blunted when insulin resistance is high.

Stimulation of thermogenesis has been one approach to the treatment of obesity from a time more than 100 years ago when thyroid extract was first used. Although thyroid hormones increase energy expenditure and reduce body fat, they also increase the loss of lean body mass and bone calcium. If these effects could be eliminated, the thermogenic effect and loss of fat might be beneficial. The use of dinitrophenol, a thermogenic drug that uncouples oxidative phosphorylation, produced weight loss but had the highly undesirable side-effect of producing cataracts and neuropathy.

β_3-Adrenergic receptor agonists have been evaluated in clinical programs by several pharmaceutical companies. Such drugs have the potential to increase energy expenditure. Previous versions of β_3-agonists did not meet with success in clinical trials, largely due to lack of specificity and potency for the human β_3-receptor. Within the next few years, the improved β_3-agonists currently being developed should address whether or not this is a viable strategy.

The original brown fat uncoupling protein (UCP1) has a well-established role in rodent temperature and body weight regulation. Increased expression and/or activation of this protein uncouples oxidative phosphorylation, resulting in the conversion of energy to heat (thermogenesis). The importance of this molecule in humans has always been questioned due to the very low levels of brown fat (and hence UCP1 expression) in adult humans. Recently, the identification of two additional uncoupling proteins (UCP2 and UCP3) that are highly expressed in adult human thermogenic tissues has attracted considerable interest. It is possible that drugs activating or increasing the expression of UCP2 and UCP3 would have important effects on energy expenditure.

Obesity is a reflection of increased fat stores, in both subcutaneous and visceral fat deposits. The obese individual has enlarged or hypertropic fat cells that can be viewed as the pathology of obesity. The many products made and secreted from fat cells play an important role in the pathogenic consequences of obesity. The control of the processes of fat synthesis, deposition and mobilization are all important components of the controlled system. Insulin plays an important role in the activation of lipogenesis in fat cells. It also inhibits lipolysis and is involved in fat cell differentiation.

The differentiation of fat cells has several steps and requires a number of factors, in addition to insulin, to complete the process. One of the early steps involves fatty acids interacting with the peroxisome proliferator-activated receptor-γ (PPAR-γ). This PPAR-γ forms a heterodimer with the retinoid X receptor (RXR) to initiate the process of fat cell differentiation. Activation of the process will increase fat cell differentiation, and inhibition of RXR will inhibit this process. Manipulation of the PPAR-γ system offers a tantalizing process for control of fat cell differentiation.

The enzyme protein tyrosine phosphatase-IB (PTP-1B) has been implicated in insulin resistance. Recently, it has been demonstrated that, in PTP-1B knockout mice, insulin resistance is reduced, yet the mice appear otherwise healthy. Of interest for obesity is that these mice do not become obese when eating a high fat diet. The reason for the protection from diet-induced obesity is currently unknown. Nevertheless, these data suggest that inhibiting PTP-1B activity may have potential for modulating obesity.

Enzymes involved in fat metabolism may be important in obesity. A notable example is the recently identified acyl CoA : diacylglycerol transferase (DGAT), the enzyme responsible for the final step in the glycerol phosphate pathway of triglyceride synthesis. Proteins involved in adipocyte differentiation, angiogenesis or apoptosis could also be targeted as a way to reduce fat mass. However, for each of these potential targets, it must be demonstrated that the reduced ability to synthesize or store fat is sensed by the body and translated into decreased energy intake or increased energy expenditure. Otherwise, the inability to deliver excess calories to adipose tissue could have serious secondary consequences as lipids accumulate in the blood or various organ systems.

AFFERENT SIGNALS

- There is a fatty acid receptor in the tongue acting through the potassium rectifier channel

- Gastrointestinal peptides such as cholecystokinin, ghrelin or enterostatin may be afferent satiety signals

- Pancreatic peptides such as glucagon-like peptide-1 may be a satiety signal

- Fatty acid digestion and fatty acid oxidation may also be a satiety signal

- Leptin is a key afferent signal from the fat cell

- A dip in plasma glucose precedes more than 50% of meals

Information generated during metabolism and from the external environment both provide signals that play a role in the control of feeding. The external signals from sight, sound and smell are all distance signals for identifying food or danger if food is sought.

The oral and nasal cavity are the first lines of exposure to food stuffs. Taste and smell can produce important positive and negative feedback signals. The recent discovery of taste and smell receptors for polyunsaturated fatty acids on the taste bud, which modulate a potassium rectifier channel, offers a new opening into modifying taste inputs into the food intake system.

Gastrointestinal peptides have long been studied as regulators of satiety. All of these peptides reduce food intake except ghrelin. Ghrelin is a small peptide produced in the stomach that interacts with the growth hormone secretogogue receptor to enhance feeding. Current studies suggest that ghrelin may play an important meal-to-meal role in the regulation of feeding. An antagonist to ghrelin would be interesting as a potential agent for the treatment of obesity. Cholecystokinin (CCK), like the rest of the intestinal peptides, inhibits food intake in animals and human beings. Peptide analogs of CCK have been developed, but none have reached the clinic. Gastrin-inhibitory peptide (also called glucose–insulin peptide) reduces food intake and stimulates insulin secretion. If the duration of action of these inhibitory peptides could be increased by blocking their breakdown, or if effective analogs could be developed, they would have the potential to reduce food intake clinically.

Pancreatic peptides also modulate feeding. Both glucagon and its 6–29 amino acid derivative, glucagon-like peptide-1 (GLP-1), reduce food intake in animals and man. Analogs or small molecules that might influence GLP-1 receptors, GLP-1 release or duration of action would be interesting candidates to treat obesity or diabetes. Enterostatin, the pentapeptide signal portion of pancreatic co-lipase, is of interest because it selectively reduces fat intake in experimental animals. This peptide increases satiety in human beings and reduces food intake in baboons. Here again, a small peptide analog could be useful as a strategy for reducing intake of single meals.

The successful introduction of orlistat to the market has demonstrated that drugs that inhibit the digestion of dietary fat can be an important component of anti-obesity therapy. However, side-effects of orlistat, resulting from fecal fat loss, can be a problem for some patients. The weight loss associated with use of orlistat when given with meals indicates that use of a short-acting medication with meals is sufficient to reduce food intake and body weight. This would suggest that some of the other short-term agents discussed here might serve as satiety signals for reducing body weight, and that could be used meal by meal when needed.

Nutrients may also be afferent satiety signals. Pyruvate, lactate and 3-hydroxybutyrate all reduce food intake when injected into experimental animals. Hydroxycitrate found in plants (*Garcinia cambogia*) interacts with citrate : ATP lyase and has been shown to reduce food intake in animals, but not in human beings.

Leptin is the best known of the afferent fat signals and the best candidate for the primary signal communicating body fat information to the central nervous system. Identification of this peptide through positional cloning in 1994 provided major new insights into the regulation of food intake, energy expenditure and body fat. It is now clear that this cytokine derived primarily from fat cells, but also from the placenta and possibly the stomach, reduces food intake and increases the activity of the thermogenic components of the sympathetic nervous system. Modulation of neurons in the arcuate nucleus by leptin results in reduced secretion of neuropeptide Y (NPY) and agouti-related protein (AGRP) and increased secretion of pro-opiomelanocortin (POMC; the precursor of α-melanocyte-stimulating hormone (α-MSH) that reduces food intake) and the peptide product of cocaine–amphetamine-regulated transcript (CART). Because of these coordinated effects of leptin, this adipocyte-derived cytokine has been used in a clinical trial where there was a dose-related weight loss, but with significant discomfort at the injection site. It has also been shown to be clinically effective in those rare individuals who lack leptin and to almost completely eliminate body fat in a transgenic mouse that over-expresses leptin. Despite the limited effect of leptin in this early clinical trial, there is still great potential for a leptin-like product or a drug that can activate the intracellular signalling system modulated by leptin. The development of small molecule agonists for the leptin receptor remains a viable idea. These could be both orally available and able to penetrate the blood–brain barrier, thereby allowing much more potent stimulation of the leptin receptor than a protein limited by saturable transport across the blood–brain barrier. Alternatively, sensitizers of the leptin pathway could be developed, as is now occurring with insulin sensitizers in type 2 diabetes. Ciliary neurotropic factor (CNTF) is a neurocytokine that is expressed in glial cells and reduces food intake and body weight in rodents, possibly through the activation of the Janus kinase/signal translation and transduction (JAK/STAT) pathway in leptin receptor-expressing cells. Although CNTF is unlikely to be involved in normal body-weight regulation, the potential pharmacological utility of this cytokine is being tested.

A dip in the circulating level of glucose precedes the onset of eating in more than 50% of the meals in animals and human beings. When this dip is blocked, food intake is delayed. The pattern recognized by this dip is independent of the level from which the drop in glucose begins. The small drop in glucose continues even when food is not available. The dip follows a small rise in insulin, suggesting that insulin stimulates the fall in glucose.

THE CENTRAL CONTROLLER

- Feeding is integrated in the medial hypothalamus

- Monoamines including norepinephrine, serotonin, dopamine and histamine modulate feeding

- Neuropeptides can increase or decrease feeding

- Neuropeptide Y, and the agouti-related peptide acting through MC4 receptors, melanin concentrating hormone (MCH), ghrelin, orexin and opioids stimulate feeding

- α-MSH, cocaine–amphetamine-regulated transcript (CART), and corticotropin releasing hormone decrease feeding

In recent years, the most intensively explored areas of food intake regulation have been the analysis of central monoamine and neuropeptide mechanisms. The serotonin system has been the most heavily studied of the monoamine pathways and serotonin receptors modulate both the quantity of food and macro-nutrient selection. Stimulation of the serotonin receptors in the paraventricular nucleus reduces fat intake, with little or no effect on the intake of protein or carbohydrate. The reduction in fat intake by fenfluramine is probably through 5-HT_{2C} receptors, since its effect is attenuated in 5-HT_{2C} knockout mice. Accordingly, specific 5-HT_{2C} agonists may be important future therapeutics. Serotonin receptors may be effective sites for modulation of both total intake and fat intake. However, the unfortunate development of valvulopathy with fenfluramine and dexfenfluramine will surely provide a damper on further efforts at new drug development using serotonin receptors.

The stimulation of α_1-noradrenergic receptors reduces food intake. Phenylpropanolamine is an α_1-agonist that has a modest effect on food intake. Some of the antagonists to the α_1 receptors that are used to treat benign prostatic hypertrophy produce weight gain, indicating that this receptor is clinically important. Stimulation of α_2 receptors will increase food intake in experimental animals, and a polymorphism in the $\alpha_{2\beta}$ adrenoceptor has been associated with reduced metabolic rate in humans. On the other hand, the β_2 receptors in the brain reduce food intake. These receptors can be activated by agonist drugs, by releasing norepinephrine in the vicinity of these receptors, or by blocking the reuptake of norepinephrine.

Stimulation of dopamine receptors can also reduce food intake. Both the D-1/D-5 and the D-2/D-3,4 receptors appear to have this effect. However, they also influence the preference for foods and the hedonic experiences surrounding food. Whether they offer effective approaches to treatment of obesity remains to be determined.

Pharmacologically defined central histamine receptors have also been identified experimentally as modulators of feeding. Recently, the histamine H_3 receptor molecule has been identified and this should enable more detailed studies of the role of H_1 receptors in body-weight regulation. It is conceivable that some of the weight gain seen with the broad-based phenothiazines may result from their interaction with histaminergic receptors. The effects of histamine may be through its effect on release of norepinephrine.

The number of neuropeptides shown to affect food intake has been growing in recent years at an accelerating rate. However, the degree of biological validation and likely relative importance vary considerably. Neuropeptide Y is among the most potent stimulators of feeding. Its synthesis and release is modulated by insulin, leptin and starvation. Antagonists to either the Y-5 or the Y-1 NPY receptor could be explored as potential agents for treatment of obesity. The fact, that NPY, NPY Y-1 and NPY Y-5 receptor knockouts do not affect nutrient status may imply that redundant systems can replace NPY when it is absent. This may also limit the use of potential NPY antagonists.

The melanocortin receptor system is an attractive target. A natural agonist, α-MSH, reduces food intake, and human beings and a mouse lacking POMC, the precursor of α-MSH, are obese. The biological importance of this receptor system became clear when it was shown that MC4 receptor knockout mice became massively obese, approaching the weight of the leptin-deficient obese mouse. This suggests that specific MC4 receptor agonists may become important obesity therapeutics. The melanocortin-receptor system is the one on which the genetic defect in the agouti locus of the yellow mouse plays out its role.

Antagonists to melanin concentrating hormone (MCH) receptor are another potential approach for drug development. MCH is produced by neurons in the lateral hypothalamus and microinjection of this peptide increases food intake. MCH knockout mice are lean, suggesting that the peptide has a physiological role in the control of food intake and body fat stores. The MCH receptor has recently been identified, allowing more rapid progress in this field.

The opioid receptors were the first group of peptide receptors shown to modulate feeding. They also affect macronutrient selection by modulating fat intake. Both the mu and kappa receptor can affect feeding, but whether this strategy can be applied to development of new drugs because of the linguistic connotations of 'opioid-like' is uncertain.

Several other peptides that stimulate food intake are of lesser interest because they have been associated with other significant biological events. Galanin is the first example. Mice lacking galanin are unable to maintain lactation, suggesting that modulation of milk-producing hormones may be the primary role for this peptide. Orexin A was recently identified as a peptide that stimulates food intake, but it is also deficient in dogs with narcolepsy. Thus the orexin peptide, which is abundant in the lateral hypothalamus, may serve an arousal function with feeding as one part. Whether sleepiness is a good alternative to eating is debatable. CRH and the closely related urocortin have been shown to have effects on food intake and body weight. The CRH receptors and CRH binding protein have therefore been considered as anti-obesity targets. However, intervention with this pathway may have negative consequences on the stress axis and anxiety.

EFFERENT SIGNALS

- Growth hormone, testosterone and estrogen affect the distribution of body fat

- Glucocorticoids modulate body fat and participate in fat cell differentiation

- Insulin is essential for fat cell differentiation and is involved in lipogenesis and lipolysis

The motor system for food acquisition and the endocrine and autonomic nervous systems are the major efferent control systems involved with acquiring food and regulating body fat stores. Among the endocrine controls are growth hormone, thyroid hormone, gonadal steroids (testosterone and estrogens), glucocorticoids and insulin.

During growth, growth hormone and thyroid hormone work together to increase growth of the body. At puberty, gonadal steroids enter the picture and lead to shifts in the relationship of fat to lean body mass in boys and girls. Testosterone increases lean mass relative to fat and estrogen has the opposite effect. Testosterone levels fall when human males grow older, and there is a corresponding increase in visceral and total body fat and a decrease in lean body mass. This may be compounded by the decline in growth hormone that is also associated with an increase in fat relative to lean mass. Both testosterone and growth hormone have been used to treat obesity. Growth hormone increases energy expenditure and increases the loss of fat. Growth hormone also reduces visceral fat more than total fat. Testosterone and anabolic steroids in males can lower visceral fat relative to total body fat, suggesting selective effects on different fat deposits. At high doses both testosterone and growth hormone have undesirable side-effects. Testosterone is related to the development of prostatic hypertrophy and prostatic cancer. Excess growth hormone, on the other hand, has been associated with enhanced risk of cardiovascular disease. The local injection or topical application of lipolytic drugs has also been reported to have modest effects in reducing local fat deposits. This cosmetic effect could be particularly appealing to some individuals.

Glucocorticoids are critical for the development of obesity. In all forms of experimental obesity, glucocorticoids are necessary for the development and maintenance of obesity. Adrenalectomy in animals with a lesion in the ventromedial hypothalamus (VMH) reverses the obesity. In genetically obese animals, adrenalectomy stops the progression, but does not reverse the syndrome. In human beings, excess production of glucocorticoids produces modest obesity, and destruction of the adrenal glands is associated with loss of body fat. Recent data suggest that 11-β-hydroxy steroid dehydrogenase in visceral fat may regulate the amount of cortisol, relative to cortisone, and thus the quantity of visceral fat.

Insulin is essential for the development of obesity. It plays a key role in lipogenesis and inhibition of lipolysis. Destruction of the beta-cells in experimental forms of obesity slows or arrests its development. Absence of insulin, seen in type 1 diabetics, is associated with normal body weight. Treatment of diabetics with insulin, or drugs that increase insulin secretion from the beta-cell, increase body fat relative to other forms of treatment for diabetes.

The autonomic nervous system is the other major regulator of internal metabolism. The efferent parasympathetic (vagal) system modulates gastric emptying, hepatic metabolism and insulin secretion, among other controls. The sympathetic nervous system, on the other hand, modulates thermogenesis, insulin secretion and vascular reactivity through regionally controlled effects on blood vessels. In a variety of experimental studies, there is a strong reciprocal relationship between food intake and the thermogenic component of the sympathetic nervous system. Clinical studies with a thermogenic drug combination of ephedrine and caffeine show that more than half of the weight loss results from a decrease in food intake. This suggests that drugs which modulate thermogenesis may also have important effects on food intake.

From this brief review of the control of energy balance and some of its underlying mechanisms, it is an easy transition to selecting potential targets for development of anti-obesity drugs. Which of these drug targets will be the most potent and have the easiest development phase cannot be predicted ahead of time.

3

Treatment of obesity

HISTORICAL PERSPECTIVE

- Thyroid extract was first used over 100 years ago

- Dinitrophenol was used briefly until cataracts and neuropathy developed

- D-Amphetamine was introduced in the 1930s but was addictive

- After World War II, thyroid, digitalis, diuretics and D-amphetamine became popular as the 'Rainbow Pills', until deaths were reported

- The appetite suppressant, aminorex, produced pulmonary hypertension, leading to its withdrawal in the early 1970s

- Very low calorie diets, including the 'Last Chance Diet' were popular, although deaths were reported when the diets contained poor-quality protein

- Valvulopathy was reported in patients treated with fenfluramine/phentermine

- Phenylpropanolamine produced strokes in women and was withdrawn

In this chapter, there follows an account of the growth of pharmacotherapy for obesity. I will trace both the introduction of new ideas and the unfortunate outcome that many of them have produced. It is this string of 'unintended consequences', leading to deaths and disability, that must give pause in future drug development. This sensitivity to the 'law of unintended consequences', along with the stigma that confronts treatment of obesity, make it a challenge to convince the Regulatory Agencies and the medical profession that it is better to treat the overweight

patient than to wait until the associated conditions develop and treat them individually.

The beginning of 'modern' pharmacotherapy for obesity can be dated to 1893 when the use of *thyroid extract* was first reported. This crude preparation produced weight loss and its use has continued almost to the present time. It soon became clear, as methods for measuring metabolic expenditure were developed, that this hormone increased energy expenditure. The use of thyroid extract could be justified because the 'metabolic rate' of many overweight people was said to be 'low'. It was widely believed that their low metabolism was the cause of obesity and that using a metabolic stimulant would 'correct' the problem. As the methodology improved, it has become clear that overweight people have higher metabolic rate that is directly related to the size of the fat free mass. The earlier concept of a low metabolic rate was due to the correction of oxygen consumption for body weight that produced an artificially low result.

The next important development was the introduction of *dinitrophenol* in the late 1920s. This therapy was based on the observation that people working with dinitrophenol in the chemical dye industry often lost weight. When the drug was tried in human beings, it produced weight loss, but was also associated with significant side-effects such as neuropathy and cataracts. Although this drug has not been used for nearly 50 years, it has an interesting potential mechanism of 'uncoupling' oxidative phosphorylation.

Shortly after the disappearance of dinitrophenol, *amphetamine* was introduced, based on the observations that patients with narcolepsy who were treated with dextro-amphetamine lost weight. However, amphetamine was addictive. This addictive property of D-amphetamine, biphetamine and methamphetamine has given the whole class of appetite suppressant drugs a negative halo, under which new appetite suppressants continue to suffer. Amphetamine is an alpha-methyl derivative of β-phenylethanolamine and its name is derived from alpha-methyl-β-phenethylamine. The backbone for amphetamine served as the structure for many chemical derivatives that were marketed over the next 25 years, including phentermine, diethylpropion, phenmetrazine, phendimetrazine and benzphetamine. All of these drugs have been classified as potentially addictive by the US Drug Enforcement Agency (DEA).

The most interesting derivative of this class was *fenfluramine*. This compound has a tri-fluoromethyl moiety in the meta-position of the phenyl ring. This substitution completely changes the pharmacology of the β-phenethylamine backbone. Fenfluramine is a drug that works by releasing serotonin and partially blocking its reuptake into the pre-synaptic nerve ending. The nor-fenfluramine metabolite is also active and is thought to function as a direct serotonin receptor agonist. Fenfluramine was introduced in 1972 in both Europe and the United States. Even though there was no clear evidence of addictive potential, it was given a Schedule IV listing by the DEA of the US Government because it is a β-phenethylamine. Just prior to its withdrawal in 1997, this drug was about to be descheduled because there was no evidence of addictive potential demonstrated during its 25 years of use. One of the interesting side-effects of fenfluramine was the potential for depression when it was withdrawn.

The only drug approved for treatment of obesity that was not a derivative of β-phenethylamine was mazindol, a tricyclic compound. This drug was initially developed in a screen for antidepressant drugs, but proved to have appetite-suppressant properties. This connection between antidepressant drugs and fat stores is a recurring theme. Mazindol is a norepinephrine reuptake inhibitor without known abuse potential, but it is nonetheless a DEA Schedule IV drug. It was marketed in 1974, but is no longer sold.

After the last of this older generation of drugs was approved, the use of very low calorie diets began its rapid growth. It reached a peak in the early 1980s with the Cambridge Diet and the Optifast program. A side-effect of this diet plan was the 'Last Chance Diet', a popular book touting the very low calorie diet, which used poor-quality protein and was accompanied by a rash of deaths in the late 1970s. When the quality of the protein in these diets was improved, they became much safer. Paralleling the rise in the use of the very low calorie diets was the introduction of popular franchised weight loss programs such as that by Jenny Craig. However, the furor over these deaths led to another set of Congressional hearings similar to the ones following the deaths from the Rainbow pills nearly 20 years earlier.

The fact that fenfluramine, as a serotonergic drug, produced weight loss led to trials of newer serotonergic drugs as possible weight loss agents. Fluoxetine in its early clinical trials was shown to produce weight loss, and these trials showed that there was a dose-related decrease in body weight of modest degree. However, with continued therapy, the weight loss stopped and weight was regained, returning to nearly normal levels, even in the presence of continued therapy. This is the only example of loss of therapeutic efficacy with continued medication among appetite-suppressant drugs.

At the same time as fluoxetine was being tested, the β_3-adrenergic receptor was identified as a thermogenic target. Using rodent adipose tissue as a screen, drugs that stimulated the β_3 receptor were developed and tested in human beings. The β_3-adrenergic agonists were thermogenic, but also produced tremors and required multiple dosing schedules. None have gone into a multi-center clinical trial. After the β_3 receptor was cloned, the differences between the human and rat receptors were recognized, and a new generation of compounds are currently under development

The next chapter in this story was the development of *combination therapy*. We have already described drugs that act on noradrenergic and serotonergic receptors. It was a rational step to suggest that a combination of drugs that acted on different receptors might be better than monotherapy. Weintraub and his group tested this possibility and showed that the combination of fenfluramine plus phentermine produced a 15.9% weight loss compared to a 4.9% weight loss in the placebo-treated patients at 6 months. When these data were published in 1992, they attracted national attention and became widely used. Then came the disaster. In 1997, the *New England Journal of Medicine* violated its own injunction not to release data before they were published and permitted the authors to alert the public to the appearance of aortic valve regurgitation in some patients treated with the combination of fenfluramine and phentermine. It soon became clear that this treatment might produce valvulopathy in up to 25% or more of the treated patients. Armed with this information, fenfluramine and dexfenfluramine were removed from the market worldwide on September 15, 1997. Continuing follow-up of this group of patients has shown that some of them remit.

The final chapter in this historical saga was the publication in December 1994 of a report that leptin had been cloned. Leptin is a cytokine-like peptide produced primarily in adipose tissue. Human beings or animals lacking leptin or its functional receptor are massively obese, indicating that this peptide produces an important signal. The excitement generated by this finding, and the subsequent demonstration that a mouse lacking a functional melanocortin 4 receptor was massively obese, galvanized the search for newer therapies for obesity by the pharmaceutical industry.

MECHANISMS OF ACTION

- Reducing food intake is one strategy to treat obesity

- Altering metabolism is a second strategy

- Increasing thermogenesis is a third strategy

In the section on etiology, a number of mechanisms were discussed using a feedback model. The basic elements of this model can be used in classifying current therapies. They can be divided into three groups: treatments that reduce food intake, treatments that alter metabolism, and treatments that are thermogenic. At the present time, there are examples of each of these three mechanisms that have been applied clinically. The following section will review each of them using the currently available drugs. For more detail, the reader is referred to two reviews on this subject[1,2].

CURRENTLY AVAILABLE DRUGS

- Sibutramine uses a strategy of reducing food intake by blocking reuptake of serotonin and norepinephrine

- Orlistat uses a strategy that alters metabolism by blocking pancreatic lipase

- The combination of ephedrine and caffeine uses a thermogenic strategy, but also decreases food intake

Agents that reduce food intake

Both noradrenergic and serotonergic drugs are currrently available. The noradrenergic drugs can be divided into three groups. In the first group are those that work by releasing norepinephrine from stored granules in the neural endplate. This would include *diethylpropion, benzphetamine, phendimetrazine, phentermine* and the *amphetamines*. All of these drugs are stimulants of the central nervous system and can increase blood pressure transiently. In the United States at the present time, generic phentermine is prescribed much more often than either of the newly released drugs. These older noradrenergic drugs were evaluated for clinical effectiveness more than 30 years ago. The clinical trials were usually short term, and often used cross-over designs. In 1975, the FDA published a brief review of the new drug applications that had been submitted for this class of drugs. In almost all of the trials comparing placebo and active drug, the weight loss and percentage of patients achieving a degree of weight loss were higher for the active agent than placebo. We are only aware of one trial comparing phentermine with placebo that lasted more than 24 weeks. In this trial, phentermine, whether used continuously or intermittently, produced similar weight loss that was significantly greater than in the placebo-treated group. Recently, phentermine, diethylpropion and other drugs in this class have been removed from the market in those European countries that had permitted their use.

Phenylpropanolamine, a drug now removed from the market, is in the second group, because this drug acts directly on α_1-adrenergic receptors. Injection of this drug into the paraventricular nucleus of animals reduces food intake and can be blocked with α_1-adrenergic antagonists. The data from clinical trials suggest that the weight loss with phenylpropanolamine is about half that with the other noradrenergic drugs, but the quality of the clinical trials are not very good.

The third mechanism for noradrenergic drugs is to block reuptake of norepinephrine. *Mazindol* is the only example of this type of drug but it is no longer marketed. Mazindol is a tricyclic that was developed from an antidepressant screen and then found to have a greater effect on weight loss. Almost all of the clinical trials with this drug were performed more than 25 years ago, and most of them utilized a cross-over design that limits the interpretation of the data. In addition to its appetite-suppressant effects, there are data suggesting that this drug may produce a modest degree of 'thermogenesis' in experimental animals.

Fenfluramine and *dexfenfluramine* were the first two serotonergic drugs, but, as noted above, they were withdrawn from the market in 1997 due to their association with valvulopathy. *Fluoxetine* and *sertraline*, two highly specific serotonin reuptake inhibitors, both suffer from loss of efficacy during continued administration and have never been approved for weight loss, although they are widely used as antidepressants.

The only drug in this class approved for long-term use is *sibutramine*, that blocks the reuptake of serotonin and norepinephrine and, to a lesser degree, dopamine. Sibutramine is a sympathomimetric drug of the β-phenylethylamine class. It was initially developed as an antidepressant, but found to have a greater effect on body weight than on depression. Sibutramine produces dose-related weight loss. In two weight maintenance studies where sibutramine and placebo were randomly assigned after initial weight loss, sibutramine largely maintained or extended weight loss over what was produced by the initial weight loss strategy. Sibutamine is approved for long-term use, but is classified as a Schedule IV by the DEA, even though there is no evidence that it is addictive. There is also no evidence that sibutramine causes valvular lesions of the type seen with the combination of fenfluramine and phentermine. It is worth noting that sibutramine is very similar to the antidepressant venlafaxine. Both are serotonin–norepinephrine reuptake inhibitors and are derived from the β-phenylethylamine structure. In the package insert, weight loss is reported with venlafaxine. Here again is another example of the relationship between antidepressant and weight loss drugs.

Recently, *bupropion*, another antidepressant drug, has been shown to produce weight loss. The number of subjects was small, but the study provides another connection between antidepressants and weight loss.

Drugs that alter metabolism

Although a number of potential agents are available in this area, *orlistat* is the only one approved for treatment of obesity. Orlistat is placed in this group because it partially blocks the lipolytic effect of pancreatic lipase in the digestion of triglycerides in the intestine. On a 30% fat diet, orlistat produces a dose-dependent increase in fecal fat loss, with a plateau at about 30% of the ingested fat, which occurs at a dose of 400 mg/day. In clinical trials and in clinical use, the drug is given three times daily with meals,

at 120 mg. Several 1- and 2-year clinical trials have been published with this drug. In a trial where subjects were re-randomized at the end of 1 year, it was reported that weight loss with orlistat was about 10% below baseline at 1 year compared to a weight loss of 6% below baseline at 1 year in the placebo treated group. In subjects re-randomized to the opposite treatment, those going from placebo to orlistat lost weight and those switched from orlistat to placebo gained weight. In a clinical trial in which orlistat was introduced after weight loss had been produced by diet, the subjects randomized to orlistat regained 32% of the lost weight compared to a regain of slightly over 50% for those randomized to placebo. On this basis, orlistat is approved for long-term use and for maintenance of weight loss.

Testosterone is a second agent that has been used in clinical trials of mildly hypogonadal men. In this group, there was a significant decrease in visceral fat by increasing testosterone to the upper limits of normal. The decrease in visceral fat was significantly greater than the mobilization of total fat, suggesting a selective effect of fat mobilization. Anabolic steroids may also have this effect.

Growth hormone increases linear growth until the growth plates fuse. It also leads to a redistribution of body tissues, with a decrease in adipose tissue fat and an increase in lean tissue. In clinical trials, growth hormone, like testosterone, reduces visceral fat more than total fat.

Drugs that increase thermogenesis

There are no approved drugs for treatment of obesity that increase thermogenesis. However, *ephedrine* and *caffeine* have been tested in a double-blind clinical trial and shown to produce weight loss. Ephedrine is a propanolamine derivative that increases energy expenditure. It is available over the counter for use in asthma through its effect on β_2-adrenergic receptors. In experimental animals, stimulation of these receptors significantly reduces food intake. Ephedrine probably also acts on β_1 and β_3 receptors to produce stimulation of heart rate and oxygen consumption, respectively. A clinical trial that randomized 180 patients into four groups showed that the combination of ephedrine 20 mg and caffeine 200 mg three times daily produced a significantly greater weight loss of 16.2 kg than the 13.2 kg lost by the placebo-treated group. The groups treated with ephedrine or caffeine alone were not significantly different from the placebo group. At the end of the 6-month trial, an open-label extension was added with nearly half of the original patients receiving ephedrine and caffeine. At the end of 1 year, there was no significant difference among the original groups, and the patients on average maintained more than 10% weight loss. In metabolic studies on this combination, it was suggested that more than half of the weight loss was the result of decreased food intake and less than half due to the thermogenic effect. It is also worth noting that this combination increased the protein mass.

SIDE-EFFECTS

- Noradrenergic drugs have sympathomimetic side-effects including dry mouth, insomnia, constipation, and increases in blood pressure and heart rate

- Serotonergic drugs produce diarrhea, and may sedate, but have been associated, in some cases, with cardiac valvular regurgitation

- Orlistat produces gastrointestinal symptoms related to maldigestion of triglycerides, and it may reduce levels of fat soluble vitamins

- Ephedrine and caffeine increase blood pressure and heart rate

Noradrenergic drugs

All of the agents in this group produce insomnia, constipation and dry mouth. They all stimulate the cardiovascular system, but the magnitude of the effect is variable. For most of the drugs, the increase in heart rate and pulse is small and often returns to normal with continued therapy. The exception to this rule is sibutramine. With this drug, there is a small rise in pulse and blood pressure that lasts as long as the drug is continued. The reason why there is no tachyphylaxis to the cardiovascular effects of sibutramine, but appears to be for the other drugs in this group, is unclear, but may relate to the inhibition of the reuptake of both serotonin and norepinephrine.

Serotonergic drugs

Although fenfluramine and dexfenfluramine have been withdrawn, their side-effects are of interest. They produce dry mouth, and tend to produce diarrhea and sedative effects. Although both of these

drugs were assigned to DEA Schedule IV, there were never any documented cases of drug abuse with this compound. Its classification is an example of the negative halo effect from amphetamine and the β-phenylethylamine derivatives.

Orlistat

The major side-effects with orlistat result from the failure to digest triglyceride in the intestine due to blockade of lipase. These include anal leakage, fecal urgency, more frequent stools, staining of underwear, etc. As patients learn to use the medication, the frequency of these events, which usually occur within the first month, is sharply reduced. The other potential problem is the loss of fat-soluble vitamins in the undigested triglyceride. In the clinical studies, there was often a drop in serum vitamin levels within the normal range. Although a decrease below the normal range was unusual, it may be advisable to use a multi-vitamin supplement, taken at bedtime when it will be absorbed.

Ephedrine and caffeine

As might be expected from the mechanism of action for these drugs, the side-effects are due to stimulation of the cardiovascular system. An increase in heart rate, palpitations and a small increase in blood pressure have been observed which tend to resolve within the first month or two of treatment.

FEATURES OF AN IDEAL DRUG

- An ideal drug for obesity should be very safe
- A non-central mechanism would be preferred
- Cost will be a concern
- Both short- and long-acting drugs can be of value

There are a number of features that would be desirable for any new medication. The first is obviously safety. As we have learned over the years, the 'law of unintended consequences' can come into play after a treatment is introduced into the market place. Because obesity is a stigmatized condition, many people, particularly women, will seek any method to reduce their weight. For many of these people, there will be no clinical indication for drug therapy. If the drug works, however, as the fenfluramine/phentermine combination did, there will be an outpouring of interest in obtaining it. For this reason, drugs that are to be used for obesity must be safer than drugs for other chronic diseases.

After safety, comes efficacy. A medication must induce a greater weight loss than placebo, and for monotherapy it would be desirable to have a drug that can produce dose-related weight loss of up to 15% or more. Obviously, the greater the therapeutic effect, the greater the potential for misuse or potential side-effects. Nonetheless, a drug that only produces 5% weight loss from baseline would not be much better than a good placebo.

Mechanism of action is also important. The recent removal of sympathomimetic noradrenergic drugs from the market in Europe, and the scheduling of fenfluramine as a centrally acting weight loss medication, reflect the 'negative amphetamine halo' that may be transferred to other centrally acting drugs. Orlistat has received approval for long-term use and maintenance, whereas sibutramine only has approval for long-term use. In reality, sibutramine appears to be better at maintenance than orlistat. Thus, other things being equal, it would be better to have a peripherally acting drug than a centrally acting one.

Cost is obviously important. Because more than 20% of Americans are obese and many of them would need long-term therapy to reduce the risks of developing the associated co-morbidities, it is important to have a drug that is relatively inexpensive. If the cost of treating obesity approaches the cost of treating the co-morbidities, there will be reluctance to use this therapy. In addition, agents for treatment of obesity may need to be combined to achieve the optimal weight loss. If the agents are all expensive, this will be particularly troubling.

Whether short- or long-acting drugs are preferable is unclear. One could argue that taking a drug once a day would be beneficial. Alternatively, one could argue that taking a drug that was short-acting and that worked on a particular meal would be advantageous because then the subject could tailor the medication to their personal needs. The orlistat experience suggests the latter may indeed be a beneficial strategy.

Although diet, lifestyle and exercise are the corner stones of current cognitive approaches to treat obesity, they have been ineffective in preventing an epidemic. In this chapter, we have focused primarily on the points in a feedback model where treatments

might work. There is another model, however, that views obesity as an epidemiological disease, with food as the agent that acts on the human host to produce the disease of obesity. Some of the strategies proposed by this model are analogous to the 'tooth brush' strategies to prevent dental caries. With careful brushing of the teeth, and the use of dental floss, the development of dental disease could be dramatically reduced. However, the addition of fluoride to the water supply was far more effective in preventing dental disease, largely because it did not require individual actions such as tooth brushing to accomplish the goal. A similar line of thinking might apply to obesity. I have coined the term 'FLUORIDE hypothesis' to capture this approach to the prevention of obesity. In this context FLUORIDE becomes an acronym for the treatment and prevention of obesity: For Lowering Universal Obesity Rates Implement ideas that Do not demand Effort.

Several components of the diet may act as FLUORIDE-like agents in determining whether or not obesity develops. Breast feeding is the first example. In infants breast milk is their first food, and for many infants their sole source of nutrients for several months. There are several studies showing that breast feeding for more than 3 months significantly reduces the risk of obesity at entry into school and in adolescents when compared to infants who are breast-fed for less than 3 months. This may be an example of 'infant imprinting'. Two other examples that fall into the category of imprinting are the increased risk of obesity in offspring of diabetic mothers and in the offspring of mothers who smoked during the individual's intrauterine period.

Calcium intake is a second dietary factor that may work like FLUORIDE in reducing the development of obesity. The level of calcium intake in population studies is inversely related to the likelihood of being overweight. In other epidemiological studies and in feeding trials, higher dietary calcium levels are also associated with a reduced BMI and a reduced incidence of the insulin resistance syndrome.

The third example of dietary factors that may act like FLUORIDE is the intake of sweetened soft drinks. Soft drink consumption is a predictor of BMI in children in the Planet Health Study. A high level of soft drink consumption also predicted the increase in BMI during nearly 2 years of follow-up. Those with the highest soft drink consumption at baseline had the highest increase in BMI. As soft drink consumption in the population has increased, the consumption of milk, a major source of calcium, has decreased. When reviewing the relation of food consumption to the epidemic of obesity noted above, it became clear that the consumption of high fructose corn sweeteners increased rapidly at exactly the same time as the epidemic of obesity. The fructose that is the major sweetener in high fructose corn sweeteners differs from glucose, the other half of the sugar (sucrose) molecule in several ways. Fructose is absorbed from the GI track by a different mechanism than glucose. Glucose stimulates insulin release from the pancreas, but fructose does not. Fructose also enters muscle and other cells without depending on insulin, whereas most glucose entry into cells is insulin-dependent. Finally once inside the cell, fructose can enter the pathways that provide the triglyceride backbone (glycerol) more efficiently than glucose. Thus, a high consumption of fructose as occurs with the rising consumption of soft drinks and the use of high fructose corn sweeteners may be a 'fat equivalent'.

The FLUORIDE hypothesis suggests a number of strategies that might be implemented to reduce obesity. First, pregnant women could be encouraged not to smoke, at least not during pregnancy. Pregnant women with diabetes could also be urged to control their diabetes as carefully as possible. Third, breast feeding as the sole source of nutrition could be encouraged for at least the first 3 months after birth. Fourth, the consumption of lower fat dairy products should be encouraged during the first decades of life. Finally, the consumption of soft drinks sweetened with high fructose corn sweeteners could be reduced or the use of high fructose corn sweeteners partially or completely replaced with alternative sweeteners.

In spite of the best preventive strategies some individuals will nevertheless become obese. For them effective treatments are still needed. Lifestyle, diet and exercise can be helpful, but treatments that produce larger weight losses are needed. Only two drugs are currently approved for long-term use. More are needed. Surgical intervention for those at highest risk may also offer an effective strategy. Thus, both a feedback model and an epidemiological model are helpful in understanding and combating obesity.

REFERENCES

1. Bray GA, Greenway FL. Current and potential drugs for treatment of obesity. *Endocr Rev* 1999;20:805–75
2. Bray GA, Tartaglia LA. Medicinal strategies in the treatment of obesity. *Nature* 2000;404:672–7

Section II   Obesity Illustrated

List of Illustrations

ENCOUNTER WITH THE OBESE PATIENT

Figure 1.1
Daniel Lambert the Great was one of the largest men in recorded history

PROCEDURES TO ESTIMATE BODY COMPOSITION

Figure 1.2
Different methods by which to measure obesity

Figure 1.3
Body mass index (BMI) can be determined from this table

Figure 1.4
Classification of overweight and obesity by body mass index (BMI), waist circumference and associated disease risk

Figure 1.5
The five levels of body composition: whole body, tissue and organ system, cellular, molecular and atomic

Figure 1.6
(a) A dual x-ray absorptiometer with a patient being scanned; (b) the picture that is obtained when the scan is completed and the various compartments that can be determined; (c) an underwater weighing compartment with load cells that determine the weight of the subject when submerged

Figure 1.7
Methods of measuring body composition

Figure 1.8
Longitudinal scan of the whole body by CT scan

Figure 1.9
CT scans comparing visceral versus subcutaneous fat

Figure 1.10
Fat and lean compartments of the body in obese and lean subjects, showing the relative amount of energy in each one

FACTORS AFFECTING BODY COMPOSITION

Figure 1.11
Age affects the percentage of body fat

Figure 1.12
Age also affects fat distribution

Figure 1.13
Ethnicity, age and gender affect the percentage of body fat

Figure 1.14
Socioeconomic status can also affect body composition

PREVALENCE

Figure 1.15
The weight of American men inducted into the army, for a given height depicted versus time since the American Civil War (1861–5)

Figure 1.16
Prevalence of obesity in children in the United States

Figure 1.17
The prevalence of obesity in the USA in (a) 1991 and (b) 1998

Figure 1.18
Prevalence of obesity in adults in the United States

Figure 1.19
Differences in prevalence of obesity (body mass index > 30) in men and women among ethnic groups in the United States

Figure 1.20
Increasing prevalence of obesity over time (body mass index > 30) in different countries around the world

GENETIC FACTORS

Figure 2.1
A model showing the relationship of various factors associated with the control of body fat

Figure 2.2
Genetic factors are clearly involved in the development of obesity

Figure 2.3
Single-gene defects in animals have contributed enormously to our understanding of the rare human disorders

A MODEL FOR REGULATING ENERGY BALANCE

Figure 2.4
The development of obesity can be viewed as a defect in the relationship between food that is eaten and the energy that is expended

Figure 2.5
Peptides and monamines affect food intake

Figure 2.6
Reciprocal relationship of the sympathetic nervous system that is also involved in food intake

Figure 2.7
One important timing mechanism for meals may be a dip in the glucose level

FOOD INTAKE

Figure 2.8
Daily food intake is variable

Figure 2.9
Food intake changes with age

Figure 2.10
Dietary fat plays a role in the development of obesity

Figure 2.11
High fructose corn sweeteners

ENERGY EXPENDITURE

Figure 2.12
Food for a family of four for one year

Figure 2.13
In human beings, energy expenditure measured in the metabolic chamber is best represented by the fat-free body mass

Figure 2.14
Energy expenditure can be measured by administering double-labled water

Figure 2.15
Diagram showing the average energy expenditure for 10 individual women determined by doubly-labeled water

Figure 2.16
Thermic effect of food

Figure 2.17
Uncoupling proteins

FAT CELL

Figure 2.18
The fat cell is a complex hormonally regulated cell

Figure 2.19
Leptin is probably the most important circulating peptide produced by the fat cell

Figure 2.20
All you ever wanted to know about leptin but were afraid to ask

Figure 2.21
Development of the white fat cell

IMPACT ON LIFE EXPECTANCY

Figure 3.1
Conditions associated with obesity

Figure 3.2
Costs associated with obesity

Figure 3.3
A higher body weight or body mass index (BMI) increases the risk of death

Figure 3.4
The detrimental effect of obesity on longevity continues over many years

Figure 3.5
An increase in central fat also increases the risk of mortality and of several diseases

Figure 3.6
Weight gain in both men and women after the age of 18–20 years is associated with increased mortality and with an increase in the risk of several diseases

Figure 3.7
Physical fitness also impacts on the health risks of an individual

Figure 3.8
The risks for many diseases differ by ethnic groups

HEALTH RISKS ASSOCIATED WITH ENLARGEMENT OF FAT CELLS

Figure 3.9
The fat cell is an endocrine cell, and part of an endocrine organ that is widely dispersed

Figure 3.10
Weight gain precedes the onset of diabetes

Figure 3.11
A higher body mass index (BMI) is associated with a higher risk of diabetes

Figure 3.12
Central obesity increases the risk of diabetes

Figure 3.13
Weight loss improves the metabolic variables associated with diabetes

Figure 3.14
A pathophysiological model can relate the changes in fatty acid secretion to the altered responses that lead to diabetes and insulin resistance

Figure 3.15
Syndromes of insulin resistance

Figure 3.16
Obesity and risk for cardiovascular disease

Figure 3.17
The body mass index is related to the risk of heart disease

Figure 3.18
Body mass index is also related to higher levels of total cholesterol, triglycerides and systolic blood pressure and to a decreased level of HDL-cholesterol which are risk factors for disease

Figure 3.19
This figure shows a pathophysiological model of how the changes in these risk factors might develop as a result of increased levels of free fatty acids (FFA)

Figure 3.20
Visceral or central obesity, here measured by CT scans, is related to abnormal levels of lipids

Figure 3.21
Weight loss reduces total cholesterol and raises HDL-cholesterol

Figure 3.22
Body mass index, cholesterol and diastolic blood pressure each show a similar curvilinear relation with mortality rates

Figure 3.23
Weight loss reduces blood pressure over the first 2–4 years, but with longer maintenance of weight loss there is a recovery of blood pressure to normal levels

Figure 3.24
A pathophysiological model for the risk of developing hypertension

Figure 3.25
The relationship of body mass index to the risk of cancer

Figure 3.26
A pathophysiological model for risk of breast and uterine cancer in obese post-menopausal women

Figure 3.27
The relation of the increasing body mass index to the risk for gall bladder disease

Figure 3.28
A pathophysiological model for the metabolism of cholesterol in the development of gall bladder disease

Figure 3.29
A number of endocrine complications have been associated with obesity

PROBLEMS RELATED DIRECTLY TO THE MASS OF BODY FAT

Figure 3.30
Sleep apnea is a common problem particularly in overweight men

Figure 3.31
The relationship of body mass index to the risk of developing osteoarthritis

Figure 3.32
Obesity is a stigmatized condition

Figure 3.33
The effects of obesity on psychosocial difficulties

CHILDHOOD OBESITY

Figure 3.34
Complications of childhood obesity

CLASSIFICATION AND CLINICAL TYPES OF OBESITY

Figure 4.1
A classification of obesity

Figure 4.2
Photomicrograph of fat cells from an overweight individual

Figure 4.3
A second characteristic of the fat mass is the number of fat cells

Figure 4.4
Several kinds of hypothalamic disease can cause human obesity

Figure 4.5
Hypothalamic obesity

Figure 4.6
Cushing's syndrome resulting from a basophilic adenoma of the pituitary gland was originally described by Harvey Cushing in 1932

Figure 4.7
The polycystic ovary syndrome is another endocrine disease in which obesity commonly manifests itself

Figure 4.8
As the number of receptor-specific medications has increased, several classes of them have been associated with weight gain

Figure 4.9
The weight gain reported in patients treated with sulfonyl-ureas and insulin compared to the smaller gain with metformin in the United Kingdom Prospective Diabetes Study

Figure 4.10
Pregnancy is associated with weight gain

Figure 4.11
A variety of human syndromes of obesity that parallel syndromes described in animals have been reported

Figure 4.12
Weight gain in two children that are leptin-deficient

Figure 4.13
The family tree for leptin receptor deficiency

Figure 4.14
Syndromic forms of obesity most of which include hypogonadism and mental retardation

Figure 4.15
The Prader–Willi syndrome is probably the commonest phenotypic syndrome of obesity resulting from a deletion or translocation in chromosome 15

Figure 4.16
The Barbet–Biedl syndrome is a rare genetically transmitted form of syndromic obesity

Figure 4.17
Picture and growth charts of a boy and girl who are deficient in pro-opiomelanocortin, the precursor to ACTH and α-MSH

Figure 4.18
Venus of Willendorf

EVALUATION AND INTRODUCTION TO TREATMENT

Figure 5.1
Patient encounter

Figure 5.2
Natural history

Figure 5.3
Using the relationship between mortality ratios from life insurance data on the predominantly Caucasian population we can identify pre-overweight, overweight and clinically overweight groups

Figure 5.4
The metabolic syndrome and insulin resistance are strongly related to central adiposity

Figure 5.5
NHLBI algorithm for evaluating overweight

Figure 5.6
A second algorithm for evaluating overweight

Figure 5.7
Predictors of weight gain

Figure 5.8
An algorithm to approach selection of therapy

Figure 5.9
Goals of therapy for adults

Figure 5.10
Various categories of success with weight loss programs

Figure 5.11
Using the natural history of obesity, we can divide the selection of treatments up according to stage of the problem and the age of the individual

Figure 5.12
Strategies for the treatment of children

Figure 5.13
Strategies for adolescents and adults

Figure 5.14

Strategies for older people when pre-overweight, and when preventive strategies are no longer a consideration

Figure 5.15

Weight goals for overweight women

Figure 5.16

Relationship of weight loss by various treatments to imagined weight goals

BEHAVIOR MODIFICATION

Figure 6.1

The targets of behavioral therapy in the energy balance diagram

Figure 6.2

The ABC Scheme for evaluating behavioral strategies to control obesity

Figure 6.3

Behavioral approaches that are the most useful in helping to keep weight off

Figure 6.4

Behavior therapy is now a main component of most weight loss programs

Figure 6.5

The improving success of behavioral therapy over time

Figure 6.6

To monitor the conditions that affect obesity and the behavior itself requires a process

Figure 6.7

A second approach to monitoring behavior uses forms for individual behaviors

Figure 6.8

Long-term effectiveness of behavioral skills in reducing future weight of children has been demonstrated in a ten-year study

Figure 6.9

A ten-year study of behavioral therapy in Sweden has shown that with continued treatment weight can be kept lower than baseline

Figure 6.10

The intensity of the behavioral strategies also improves weight loss

Figure 6.11

The internet is the latest tool applied to behavioral therapy

Figure 6.12

Adding a structural eating plan to a behavioral plan can also improve weight loss

Figure 6.13

Adding behavioral strategies to drug treatment also improves weight loss

Figure 6.14

Learning to control eating events takes planning

DIET

Figure 7.1

Identification of the site at which diet works to influence energy balance

Figure 7.2

A classification of diets based on energy levels

Figure 7.3

To reduce calories as a strategy to lose weight, we must have an estimate for energy needs

Figure 7.4

As part of the strategy for behavioral control, a form for recording calories and for analysing the data was developed

Figure 7.5

The nutrition label for low-fat milk

Figure 7.6

A deficit of 500 kcal/day will produce about 0.5 kg weight loss per week, depending on the individual's weight

Figure 7.7

Comparison of a balanced deficit diet and a very low calorie diet

Figure 7.8

Portion control is a good strategy to control energy intake

Figure 7.9

Weight loss with meal replacements has been studied over 4 years

Figure 7.10

Calorie counters, fat gram counters and diet books

Figure 7.11

A low-fat diet ad-lib had a slightly better effect on the prevention of weight regain after an initial weight loss than a low-calorie diet

Figure 7.12

Prolonged breast feeding can reduce the prevalence of overweight at entry into school

Figure 7.13

The rate at which glucose is released from starch can be used to calculate a 'glycemic index' (GI)

Figure 7.14

The consumption of sugar-sweetened beverages in children was associated with an increasing BMI in children suggesting increased fattening

Figure 7.15

Calcium intake and body weight

Figure 7.16

The food guide pyramid

Figure 7.17

Food groups in relation to calories

Figure 7.18

Recommended dietary intake of selected nutrients for men and women

PHYSICAL ACTIVITY: A CORNERSTONE OF TREATMENT

Figure 8.1

The relation of physical activity to the energy balance equation is shown here

Figure 8.2

The relation of physical activity and energy expenditure to the total daily energy expenditure is illustrated in this figure

Figure 8.3

Energy in food is expended in basal energy needs and in activity

Figure 8.4

People in affluent countries are relatively inactive physically

Figure 8.5

The relation of inactivity to body mass index (BMI) is shown in an epidemological study

Figure 8.6

A regular pattern of physical activity can reduce the risk of premature death

Figure 8.7

When doing aerobic activity, the heart rate rises

Figure 8.8

Excercise can increase weight loss, and the weight loss is related to the amount of the exercise

Figure 8.9

Exercise as a single modality for the treatment of obesity is not very effective

Figure 8.10

Exercise is a useful strategy for preventing weight regain

Figure 8.11

Time spent viewing television is related to the degree of overweight in children

Figure 8.12

In a school-based program children in the intervention group that reduced television watching time gained less weight than the children in the control group that did not reduce television watching

Figure 8.13

People who are successful in losing weight maintain a higher level of activity

Figure 8.14

This table shows the energy expenditure associated with some common daily activities

Figure 8.15

This figure shows the amount of energy that must be expended to maintain a weight loss in individuals who have previously lost weight

Figure 8.16

Walking is an ideal method of exercise for overweight individuals

DRUGS TO TREAT OBESITY: AN INTRODUCTION

Figure 9.1

Disappointments associated with many drugs used to treat obesity during the twentieth century

Figure 9.2

Characteristics of an ideal drug

Figure 9.3

The first law of thermodynamics can be used to identify the places where drug treatment can work

DRUGS AFFECTING FOOD INTAKE: MONOAMINES

Figure 9.4

Both the noradrenergic and serotonergic receptor systems have been the basis for drugs to treat obesity

Figure 9.5

A noradrenergic nerve synapse

Figure 9.6

A serotonergic nerve synapse

Figure 9.7

Weight loss with a noradrenergic drug

Figure 9.8

Serotonergic drugs also produce weight loss

Figure 9.9

Drugs that block selectively serotonin reuptake are a second class of serotonergic drugs that have been tried in obesity

Figure 9.10

An antidepressant that reduces body weight

Figure 9.11

Since both noradrenergic and serotonergic drugs produce weight loss it was only a matter of time before the two types of drugs were combined

Figure 9.12

This combination of drugs met with the 'law of unintended consequences'

Figure 9.13

A clinical trial of sibutramine

Figure 9.14

The second trial of sibutramine

Figure 9.15

Effect of intermittent and continuous therapy with sibutramine

Figure 9.16

Side-effects of noradrenergic and serotonergic drugs

Figure 9.17

Effect of sibutramine on blood pressure

DRUGS THAT REDUCE FOOD INTAKE: PEPTIDES

Figure 9.18

Effect of metformin on weight loss

Figure 9.19

A clinical trial of leptin

Figure 9.20

Leptin-deficient subjects

Figure 9.21

Ciliary neurotrophic factor is a second peptide that was studied in a clinical trial

Figure 9.22

Glucagon-like peptide-1 which is formed by the gut during processing of proglucagon reduces food intake when given by intravenous infusion to human subjects

Figure 9.23

A clinical trial of topiramate

DRUGS THAT MODIFY METABOLISM: LIPASE INHIBITORS

Figure 9.24

The only drug in the class of lipase inhibitors is orlistat which has been approved for marketing in most countries

Figure 9.25

A clinical trial of orlistat: a first perspective

Figure 9.26

A clinical trial of orlistat: a second perspective

Figure 9.27

A second clinical trial of orlistat

Figure 9.28

Effect of orlistat for 1 year on weight loss in diabetic patients whose diabetes was controlled primarily with sulfonylureas

Figure 9.29

As a drug that blocks pancreatic lipase, the side-effects of orlistat are predictable

Figure 9.30

The development of sibutramine and orlistat that work by different mechanisms suggested that they might be additive

Figure 9.31

Both growth hormone and testosterone decrease visceral fat

DRUGS THAT AFFECT ENERGY EXPENDITURE

Figure 9.32

Increasing the expenditure of energy by increasing the metabolism is another mechanism for drugs to treat obesity

HERBAL MEDICATIONS FOR TREATMENT OF OBESITY

Figure 9.33

Hydroxycitrate, a chemical that blocks citrate lyase, was shown to produce weight loss in animals

Figure 9.34

Herbal products that supply thermogenic products similar to ephedrine and caffeine have been tested in two clinical trials

CLINICAL USE OF DRUGS TO TREAT OBESITY

Figure 9.35
Table of medications available in the United States

Figure 9.36
Drug treatment of obesity: warning

Figure 9.37
Effect size of anti-obesity drugs

SURGICAL TREATMENT OF OBESITY: A SERIOUS BUT SUCCESSFUL TREATMENT

Figure 10.1
Operations for obesity in human beings

Figure 10.2
Energy balance diagram showing where surgical treatment has its influence

Figure 10.3
Jejunoileal bypasses were the first operations that were performed regularly for obesity

Figure 10.4
A diagram of the gastric restriction operations

Figure 10.5
A diagram of the Roux-en-Y gastric bypass operation

Figure 10.6
A diagram of the biliopancreatic operation often referred to as the Scopinaro procedure

Figure 10.7
Operative complications are common

Figure 10.8
Benefits from weight loss induced by surgery

Figure 10.9
A comparison of weight loss with the gastric bypass (GBP), the vertically banded gastroplasty (VBG) and the silastic banded gastric restrictive operation

Figure 10.10
Surgical weight reduction reduces the incident cases of diabetes, hypertension and insulin resistance during the first 2 years

Figure 10.11
The pattern of change in blood pressure over the first 6 years of the Swedish Obese Subjects study is shown

Figure 10.12
Laparoscopically placed gastric band

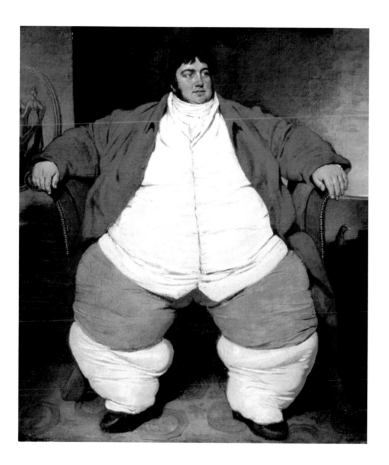

Figure 1.1 Daniel Lambert the Great was one of the largest men in recorded history. He weighed 739 lbs when he died at the age of 39 years. Many artifacts relating to his life can be found in the Leicester Museum in Leicester, UK. He is a larger-than-life example of the problems that will be the focus of this book. Reproduced with permission from The Bridgeman Art Library, London, UK

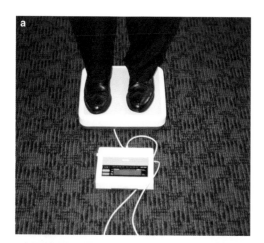

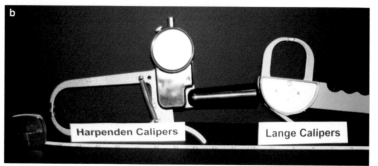

Figure 1.2 Different methods by which to measure obesity. (a) Balance; (b) skinfold calipers and tape measure

Height (inches)	Weight (pounds and kilograms)																						Height Cms
58	91	95	100	105	110	115	119	124	129	134	138	143	148	153	158	162	167	172	177	181	186	191	
	41	43	45	48	50	52	54	56	58	61	63	65	67	69	71	73	76	78	80	82	84	86	147
59	94	99	104	109	114	119	124	128	133	138	143	148	153	158	163	168	173	178	183	188	193	198	
	43	45	47	50	52	54	56	59	61	63	65	68	70	72	74	77	79	81	83	86	88	90	150
60	97	102	107	112	118	123	128	133	138	143	148	153	158	164	169	174	179	184	189	194	199	204	
	44	46	49	51	53	55	58	60	62	65	67	69	72	74	76	79	81	83	85	88	90	92	152
61	100	106	111	116	121	127	132	137	143	148	153	158	164	169	174	180	185	190	195	201	206	211	
	46	48	50	53	55	58	60	62	65	67	70	72	74	77	79	82	84	86	89	91	94	96	155
62	104	109	115	120	125	131	136	142	147	153	158	164	169	175	180	186	191	196	202	207	213	218	
	47	50	52	55	57	60	62	65	67	70	72	75	77	80	82	85	87	90	92	95	97	100	158
63	107	113	118	124	130	135	141	146	152	158	163	169	175	180	186	192	197	203	208	214	220	225	
	49	51	54	56	59	61	64	67	69	72	74	77	79	82	84	87	90	92	95	97	100	102	160
64	110	116	122	128	134	140	145	151	157	163	169	174	180	186	192	198	203	209	215	221	227	233	
	50	52	55	58	60	63	66	68	71	73	76	79	81	84	87	89	92	94	97	100	102	105	162
65	114	120	126	132	138	144	150	156	162	168	174	180	186	192	198	204	210	216	222	228	234	240	
	52	54	57	60	63	65	68	71	74	76	79	82	84	87	90	93	95	98	101	103	106	109	165
66	117	124	130	136	142	148	155	161	167	173	179	185	192	198	204	210	216	223	229	235	241	247	
	54	56	59	62	65	68	71	73	76	79	82	85	87	90	93	96	99	102	104	107	110	113	168
67	121	127	134	140	147	153	159	166	172	178	185	191	198	204	210	217	223	229	236	242	248	255	
	55	58	61	64	66	69	72	75	78	81	84	87	90	92	95	98	101	104	107	110	113	116	170
68	125	131	138	144	151	158	164	171	177	184	190	197	203	210	217	223	230	236	243	249	256	263	
	57	60	63	66	69	72	75	78	81	84	87	90	93	96	99	102	105	108	111	114	117	120	173
69	128	135	142	149	155	162	169	176	182	189	196	203	209	216	223	230	237	243	250	257	264	270	
	58	61	64	67	70	74	77	80	83	86	89	92	95	98	101	104	107	110	113	116	119	123	175
70	132	139	146	153	160	167	174	181	188	195	202	209	216	223	230	236	243	250	257	264	271	278	
	60	63	67	70	73	76	79	82	86	89	92	95	98	101	105	108	111	114	117	120	124	127	178
71	136	143	150	157	165	172	179	186	193	200	207	215	222	229	236	243	250	258	265	272	279	286	
	62	65	68	71	75	78	81	84	87	91	94	97	100	104	107	110	113	117	120	123	126	130	180
72	140	147	155	162	169	177	184	191	199	206	213	221	228	235	243	250	258	265	272	280	287	294	
	64	67	70	74	77	80	84	87	90	94	97	100	104	107	111	114	117	121	124	127	131	134	183
73	144	151	159	166	174	182	189	197	204	212	219	227	234	242	250	257	265	272	280	287	295	303	
	65	68	72	75	79	82	86	89	92	96	99	103	106	110	113	116	120	123	127	130	133	137	185
74	148	155	163	171	179	187	194	202	210	218	225	233	241	249	256	264	272	280	288	295	303	311	
	67	71	74	78	81	85	88	92	95	99	102	106	110	113	117	120	124	127	131	134	138	141	188
75	152	160	168	176	184	192	200	208	216	224	232	240	247	255	263	271	279	287	295	303	311	319	
	69	72	76	79	83	87	90	94	97	101	105	108	112	116	119	123	126	130	134	137	141	144	190
76	156	164	172	180	189	197	205	213	221	230	238	246	254	262	271	279	287	295	303	312	320	328	
	71	74	78	82	86	89	93	97	101	104	108	112	115	119	123	127	130	134	138	142	145	149	193
Body mass index	19	20	21	22	23	24	25	26	27	28	29	30	31	32	33	34	35	36	37	38	39	40	

Good weights — Overweight — Obese — Increasing risk →

Figure 1.3 Body mass index (BMI) can be determined from this table. The height is identified in inches or centimeters on the left- and right-hand side, respectively. Once the correct height is found, the weight in pounds or kilograms nearest to the patient's is identified by gliding along the corresponding row, and the BMI is read from the bottom of the chart in the same column as the correct weight. An example of the change in weight over the range of BMI from 20 to 30 can help to illustrate this point. For someone 175 cm tall, a BMI of 20 kg/m² is equivalent to 61 kg; a BMI of 25 kg/m² is equivalent to a weight of 77 kg and a BMI of 30 kg/m² is equivalent to a weight of 92 kg. Courtesy of George A. Bray

	BMI (kg/m²)	Obesity class	Disease risk (relative to waist circumference)	
			Normal Men ≤ 40 in (≤ 102 cm) Women ≤ 35 in (≤ 88 cm)	**Large** > 40 in (> 102 cm) > 35 in (> 88 cm)
Underweight	< 18.5		—	—
Normal	18.5 – 24.9		—	—
Overweight	25.0 – 29.9		Increased	High
Obesity	30.0 – 34.9	I	High	Very high
	35.0 – 39.9	II	Very high	Very high
Extreme obesity	≥ 40	III	Extremely high	Extremely high

Figure 1.4 Classification of overweight and obesity by body mass index (BMI), waist circumference and associated disease risk. Following the Consultation on Obesity by the World Health Organization in 1997 and the meetings of the Task Force on Clinical Guidelines for Diagnosis and Treatment of Obesity by the National Heart, Lung and Blood Institute (NHLBI), a world-wide definition of overweight and obesity was agreed. These criteria are shown in the table. Data derived from NHLBI Obesity Education Initiative Expert Panel. Clinical guidelines on the identification, evaluation and treatment of overweight and obesity in adults – the evidence report. *Obes Res* 1998; 6(Suppl. 2):51S–209S

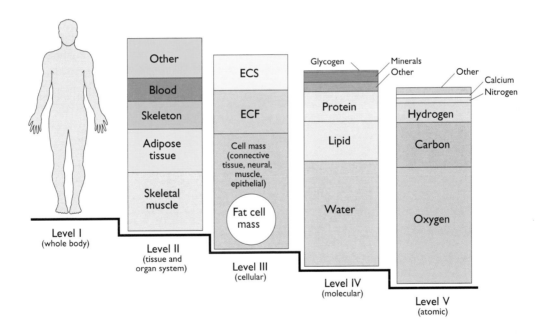

Figure 1.5 The five levels of body composition: whole body, tissue and organ system, cellular, molecular and atomic. ECS, extracellular solids; ECF, extracellular fluid. Adapted with permission of the American Journal of Clinical Nutrition from Wang ZM, Pierson RN Jr, Heymsfield SB. The five-level model: a new approach to organizing body composition research. *Am J Clin Nutr* 1992;56:19–28, © American Journal of Clinical Nutrition/American Society for Clinical Nutrition

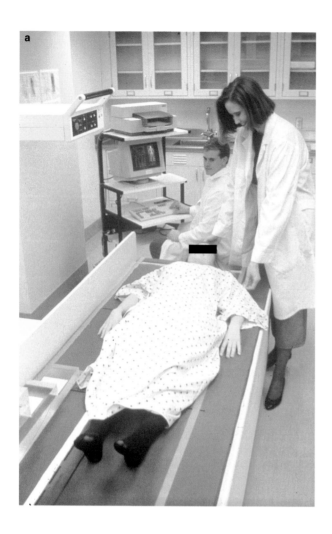

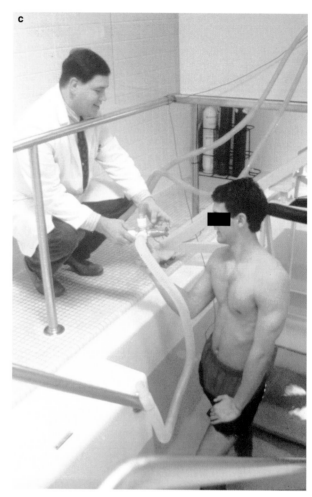

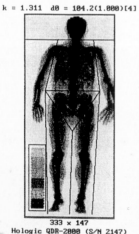

PENNINGTON BIOMEDICAL RESEARCH CENTER

333 x 147
Hologic QDR-2000 (S/N 2147)
Whole Body Version 5.40

Region	Area (cm2)	BMC (grams)	BMD (gms/cm2)
Head	258.75	610.06	2.358
L Arm	265.15	263.50	0.994
R Arm	244.36	223.64	0.915
L Ribs	135.58	93.08	0.687
R Ribs	171.57	116.17	0.677
T Spine	161.17	145.76	0.904
L Spine	49.99	53.29	1.066
Pelvis	261.15	276.78	1.060
L Leg	473.52	590.17	1.246
R Leg	464.72	583.61	1.256
TOTAL	2485.97	2956.06	1.189

Figure 1.6 (a) A dual x-ray absorptiometer with a patient being scanned; (b) the picture that is obtained when the scan is completed and the various compartments that can be determined; (c) an underwater weighing compartment with load cells that determine the weight of the subject when submerged. Lung volume is determined simultaneously with helium dilution

Method	Cost	Accuracy	Ease	Reg. fat	RAD
Anthropometry	$	M	E	Yes / No	
Densitometry	$$	H	M	No / No	
Dilution	$–$$	H	M	No / (L)	
^{40}K-counting	$$$	H	D*	No / No	
Ultrasound	$$	M	M	Yes / No	
DEXA	$$$	H	M*	Yes / L	
Impedance	$–$$	M	E	(No) / No	
Conductivity	$$$	H	D*	(No) / No	
CT scan	$$$$	H	D*	Yes / M	
MRI scan	$$$$	H	D*	Yes / No	
Neuron activation	$$$$	H	D*	No / H	

H = High; M = Moderate; L = Low; E = Easy; D = Difficult;
* = Special equipment

Figure 1.7 Methods of measuring body composition. Comparison of cost, accuracy, ease of performance and whether the procedures involve radiation and measure visceral or regional fat. CT, computed tomography; DEXA, dual energy X-ray absorptiomatry; MRI, magnetic resonance imaging

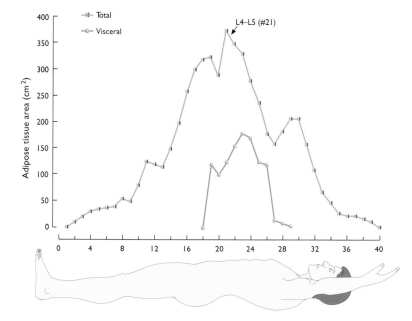

Figure 1.8 Longitudinal scan of the whole body by CT scan. The increasing level of visceral fat can be seen against the background of the skeleton. From such scans, it is possible to develop formulas for estimating compartments of body fat from other techniques. Adapted with permission from Sjostrom L, Kvist H, Cederblad A, *et al.* Determination of total adipose tissue and body fat in women by computed tomography, ^{40}K and tritium. *Am J Physiol* 1986;250: E736–45

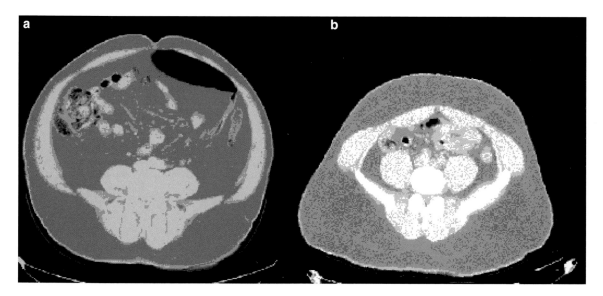

Figure 1.9 CT scans of the abdomen showing marked differences in visceral (a) and subcutaneous (b) fat in individuals with similar amounts of total fat. Courtesy of Dr. Steven Smith, Pennington Center, Baton Rouge, LA

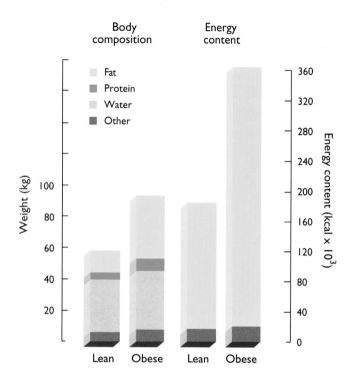

Figure 1.10 Fat and lean compartments of the body in obese and lean subjects, showing the relative amount of energy in each one. Note that a gain in weight form 60 to 90 kg increases the energy stores by almost two-fold because almost all of the extra weight is in the form of high-energy storage, i.e. fat

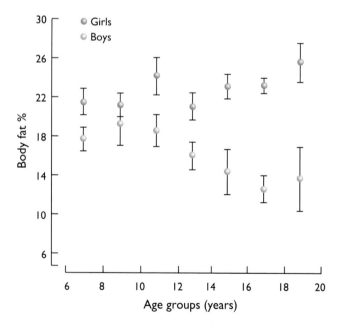

Figure 1.11 Age affects the percentage of body fat. At puberty, the percentages of body fat in boys and girls begin to diverge. This effect is due to the increase in testosterone levels in boys that causes a decrease in body fat. During adult life, the body fat content for any given body mass index is about 10–12% higher in women than in men. Adapted with permission from Molgaard C, Michaelsen KF. Changes in body composition during growth in healthy school-age children. *Appl Radiat Isot* 1998;49: 577–9

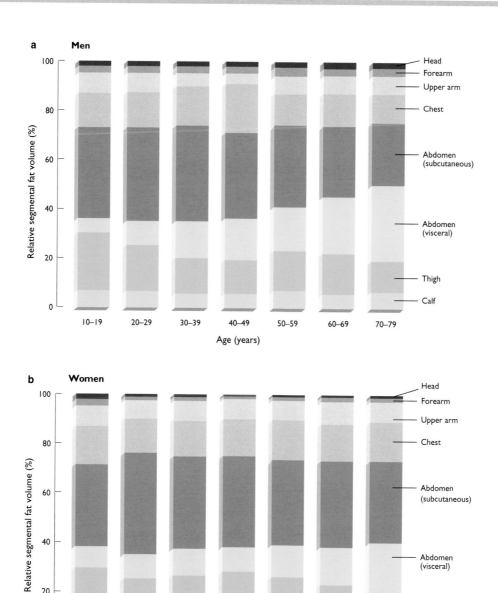

Figure 1.12 Age also affects fat distribution. This figure illustrates the changes in the amount of body fat in various compartments over the adult body by age group. (a) Men; (b) women. Adapted with permission from Kotani KK, Tokunaga K, Fujioka S, et al. Sexual dimorphism of age-related changes in whole-body fat distribution in the obese. *Int J Obes Relat Metab Disord* 1994;18:207–12

BMI	Females			Males		
	African-American	Asian	Cau-casian	African-American	Asian	Caucasian
Age 20–39						
18.5	20	25	21	8	13	8
25	32	35	33	20	23	21
30	38	40	39	26	28	26
Age 40–59						
18.5	21	25	32	9	13	11
25	34	36	35	22	24	23
30	39	41	41	27	29	29

Figure 1.13 Ethnicity, age and gender affect the percentage of body fat. For a given body mass index (BMI), the percentage of body fat differs by ethnic group. Thus, the BMI should be adjusted for the ethnicity of the individual patient. For Asians, a BMI of 23–25 is pre-obese, whereas in African-Americans the pre-obese state is a BMI of 27–29. Adapted with permission of the American Journal of Clinical Nutrition from Gallagher D, Heymsfield SB, Heo M, et al. Healthy percentage body fat ranges: an approach for developing guidelines based on body mass index. *Am J Clin Nutr* 2000;72:694–701, ©American Journal of Clinical Nutrition/American Society for Clinical Nutrition

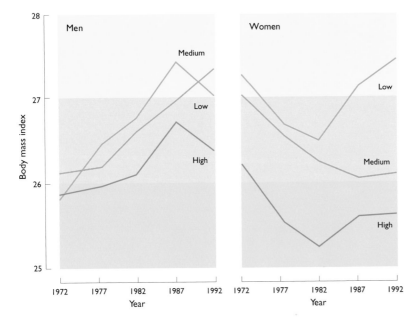

Figure 1.14 Socioeconomic status can also affect body composition. Particularly among Caucasian women, their socioeconomic status, defined by educational level and household income, influences body mass index (BMI). Women with a higher educational level, as shown in this figure, have lower BMIs than men at the same educational level in the various years of the surveys carried out by the US National Center for Health Statistics

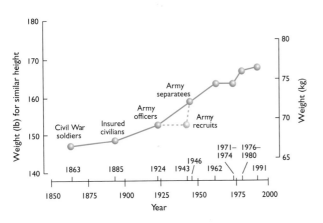

Figure 1.15 The weight of American men inducted into the army, for a given height depicted versus time since the American Civil War (1861–5). Note that there has been a steady increase in the weight for the height of 5 feet 10 inches used in this figure

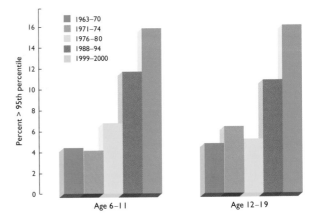

Figure 1.16 Prevalence of obesity in children in the United States. The increase in the prevalence of obesity is particularly disturbing since nearly one-third of obese adults develop their obesity in childhood. Data derived from Ogden CL, Flegal KM, Carroll MD, Johnson CL. Prevalence and trends in overweight among US Children and adolescents, 1999–2000. *J Am Med Assoc* 2002;288:1728–32

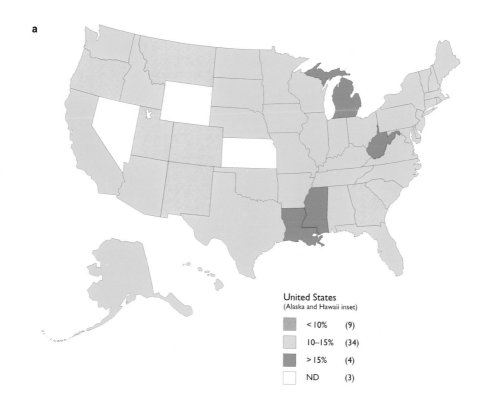

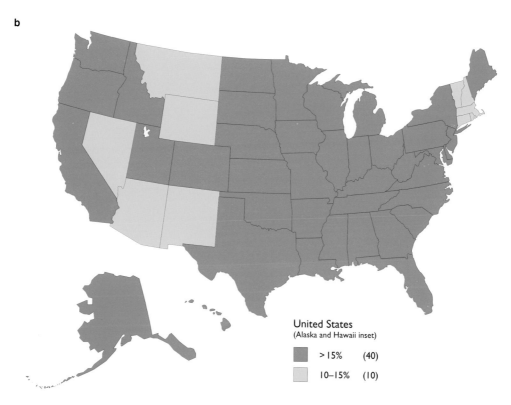

Figure 1.17 The prevalence of obesity in the USA in (a) 1991 and (b) 1998. Numbers in brackets indicate the number of American states in each category. ND, not defined

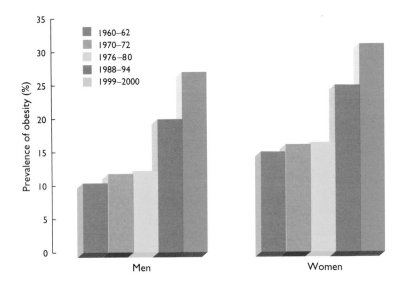

Figure 1.18 Prevalence of obesity in adults in the United States. Data derived from Ogden CL, Flegal KM, Carroll MD, Johnson CL. Prevalence and trends in overweight among US children and adolescents, 1999–2000. *J Am Med Assoc* 2002;288:1728–32

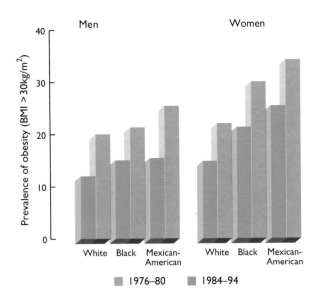

Figure 1.19 Differences in prevalence of obesity (body mass index > 30) in men and women among ethnic groups in the United States

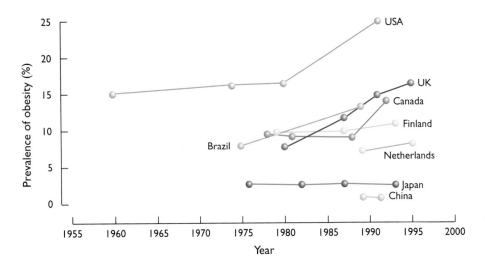

Figure 1.20 Increasing prevalence of obesity over time (body mass index > 30) in different countries around the world

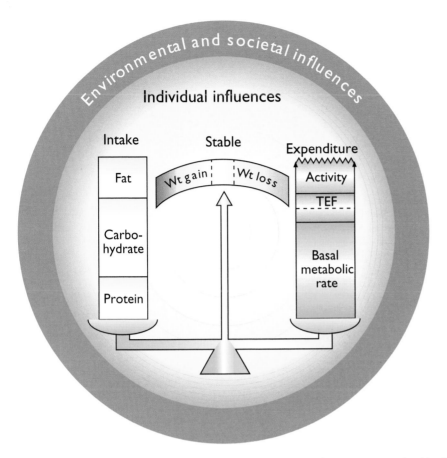

Figure 2.1 A model showing the relationship of various factors associated with the control of body fat. The individual influences include genetic background and individual choices. These collectively influence the energy balance between food intake and energy expenditure. All of these individual influences occur within the context of environmental and societal factors. TEF, thermic effect of food; Wt, weight

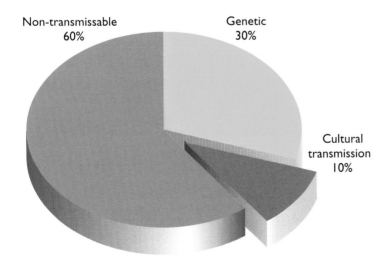

Figure 2.2 Genetic factors are clearly involved in the development of obesity. From studies of twins and adopted children, the estimate of the genetic component is around 30%; the non-genetic factors, both familial and non-familial, account for the rest. Support for the involvement of genetic factors comes from studies of nuclear families, follow-up of adopted children, and a comparison of monozygotic and dizygotic twins. Adapted with permission from Bouchard C, Perusse L, Leblanc C, et al. Inheritance of the amount and distribution of human body fat. *Int J Obes* 1988;12:205–15

Animal model	Chromosome		Human homologs	Gene defect	Gene product	Reproductive status	Mechanism
	Rodent						
Dominant inheritance							
Yellow mouse (A^{vy}; A^{sy}; A^{iy}) (gene = *agouti*)	2		20q 11.2	Agouti signaling protein (ASP) over-expressed in many tissues	ASP (131 AA with 22 AA signal peptide)	Slightly impaired	Competes with α-MSH for melanocortin receptors
Recessive inheritance							
Diabetes mouse (db = *lepr*^{db}) Fatty rat (fa = *lepr*^{fa}) Koletsky rat (fa^k = *lepr*^{k}) (gene = *lepr*)	4 5 5		1p 31	Splicing defects or extracellular deletions	Leptin receptor (505 AA)	Infertile	Impaired leptin receptor
Obese mouse (ob/ob) (gene = *lep*)	6		7q 31.3	Stop codon 105 produces truncated leptin	Leptin (167 AA)	Infertile	Leptin signal from fat to brain and other organs
Tub mouse (gene = *tub*)	7		4q 32	Splice site at 3′ coding sequence	Loss of Tub-like protein function	Impaired	Impairs neural insulin signaling
Fat mouse (gene = *cpe*^{fat})	8		11p 15	Ser 202 → Pro substitution	Carboxy-peptidase E	Impaired	Pro-hormones not cleaved

Figure 2.3 Single-gene defects in animals have contributed enormously to our understanding of the rare human disorders. This table summarizes these animal models. In Section 4, on the clinical causes of obesity, the human homologs of these animals models are described in detail

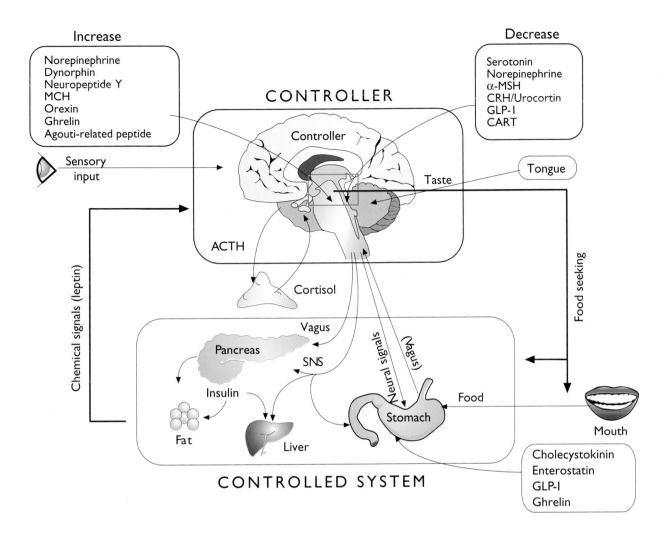

Figure 2.4 The development of obesity can be viewed as a defect in the relationship between food that is eaten and the energy that is expended. For our purposes, a feedback model will be used to show these relationships. Food intake is shown at the lower right entering the mouth. From this point through the gastrointestinal tract, signals are relayed to the brain by the vagus nerve and possibly by sympathetic nerves, as well as peptide and nutrient signals that tend to inhibit further intake of food. These signals are integrated in the brain with information from leptin produced by body fat, to activate or inhibit further eating. This central system acts on the efferent controls of feeding and seeking food. As food is digested, absorbed, metabolized or stored, internal signals from nutrient stores and glucose levels are monitored. A glucose dip occurs periodically in mammals and this may signal initiation of the next eating event. ACTH, adrenocorticotrope hormone; CART, cocaine–amphetamine-regulated transcript; CRH, corticotropin-releasing hormone; GLP-1, glucagon-like peptide I; α-MSH, α-melanocyte-stimulating hormone; MCH, melanin concentrating hormone; SNS, sympathetic nervous system

Stimulates food intake	Inhibits food intake
Agouti-related peptide	α-MSH
Dynorphin	Corticotropin-releasing hormone
Ghrelin	Cholecystokinin
Melanin concentrating hormone	Cocaine–amphetamine-regulated transcript
Neuropeptide Y	Enterostatin
Norepinephrine	Leptin
Orexin A (Hypocretin)	Glucagon-like peptide-1
	Serotonin

Figure 2.5 Peptides and monamines affect food intake. Both peptides and monoamines in the brain and in the gastrointestinal track can influence feeding. Of the peptides from the gastrointestinal track, ghrelin, cholecystokinin, enterostatin and glucagon-like peptide-1 (GLP-1) would appear to be the most important signals. Ghrelin, formed in the stomach, differs from the others by stimulating food intake. Cholecystokinin (CCK) is released into the upper intestine and reduces food intake by acting on CCK_A receptors in the pylorus, thus slowing gastric emptying. This will produce distension, which, through vagal or sympathetic afferents, can inhibit eating. Enterostatin is a pentapeptide released from pancreatic procolipase. It inhibits food intake and specifically reduces fat intake in experimental animals. GLP-1 is processed from proglucagon in the lower intestine. It inhibits food intake in lean and obese human beings. The most important peripheral signal is leptin, which is primarily produced in the adipocyte. The control of food intake within the brain involves both monoamines and peptides. Leptin is an afferent signal that acts on the arcuate nucleus to reciprocally modulate the production and release of neuropeptide Y (NPY), agouti-related peptide (Agrp), pro-opiomelanocortin (POMC) and cocaine–amphetamine-regulated transcript (CART). The first system is a stimulatory system involving NPY and Agrp. These two peptides are co-secreted and act on neuronal outputs from the paraventricular nucleus (PVN) to increase food intake. The second system involves the POMC peptide that is the precursor for α-melanocyte-stimulating hormone (α-MSH), an inhibitor of feeding, and for CART that is also an inhibitor of food intake. Afferent signals acting through the vagus nerve provide neural information from the gut to the brain. Other modulators of the γ-aminobutyric acid (GABA) output are serotonin, a monoamine that generally inhibits food intake, norepinephrine that can either inhibit or stimulate food intake, depending on where it is released, melanin concentrating hormone (MCH) that stimulates food intake, and amantadine (a cannabinoid receptor agonist) that stimulates food intake

Experimental maneuver	Changes in	
	Food intake	Sympathetic activity
Lesion in the hypothalamus VMN/PVN	↑	↓
LH	↓	↑
Peptides – Group 1 (NPY, GAL, opioids)	↑	↓
Peptides – Group 2 (CRH, BBS, CCK)	↓	↑
Chemicals – Group 1 (2-DG, NE)	↑	↓
Chemicals – Group 2 (fenfluramine, 5HT)	↓	↑

VMN, Ventromedial nucleus; PVN, paraventricular nucleus; LH, lateral hypothalamus; NPY, neuropeptide Y; GAL, galanin; CRH, corticotropin releasing hormone; BBS, bombesin; CCK, cholecystokinin; 2-DG, 2-deoxy-D-glucose; NE, norepinephrine; 5HT, serotonin

Figure 2.6 Reciprocal relationship of the sympathetic nervous system that is also involved in food intake. Norepinephrine (NE) injected into the perifornical area of the brain reduces feeding, and many of the appetite suppressants act to release or block the reuptake of norepinephrine. In animal species and in humans, a low activity of the sympathetic nervous system is associated with obesity. Moreover, a wide variety of peptides and drugs that modulate food intake have a reciprocal effect on the sympathetic nervous system

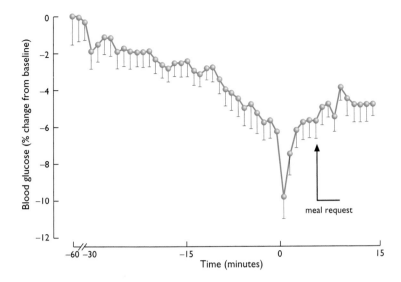

Figure 2.7 One important timing mechanism for meals may be a dip in the glucose level. This figure shows the relationship of a request for a meal to a more than 10% drop in glucose some 30 min earlier. This glucose dip occurs in both animals and man. Data derived from Campfield LA, Smith FJ, Rosenbaum M, Hirsch J. Human eating: evidence for a physiological basis using a modified paradigm. *Neurosci Biobehav Rev* 1996;20: 133–77

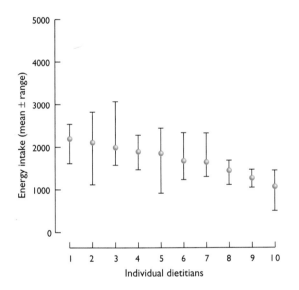

Figure 2.8 Daily food intake is variable. In this study, 10 dietitians weighed their food each day for 7 days. During this same period their energy expenditure was measured using doubly-labeled water. Each point shows the mean for one dietitian. The solid bar shows the 25th to 7th percentile of daily food intake. The upper and lower lines are the 95th percentiles for each individual. As a group the dietitians' daily food intake was within 10% of their energy expenditure. However, the variability from day to day for the same individual and between individuals is striking. Adapted with permission from Champagne CM, Bray GA, Kurtz AA, *et al*. Energy intake and energy expenditure: a controlled study comparing dietitians and non-dietitians. *J Am Diet Assoc* 2002;102:1428–32

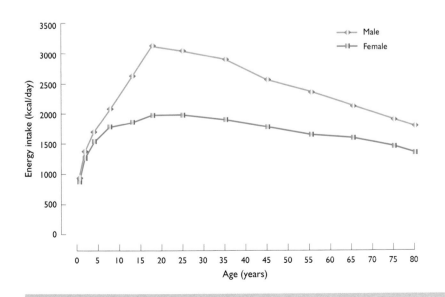

Figure 2.9 Food intake changes with age. This figure shows the integrated food intake of men and women over their life span. The data are plotted using the estimates of food intake from the National Center for Health Statistics

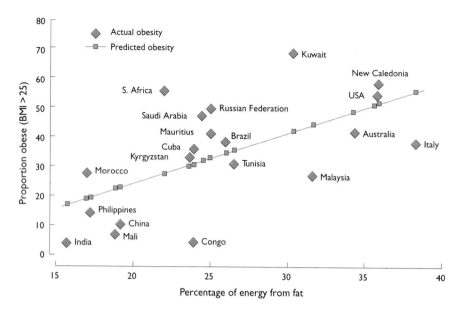

Figure 2.10 Dietary fat plays a role in the development of obesity. People in countries where the fat intake is lower are, on average, less overweight and there is less obesity. Adapted with permission of the American Journal of Clinical Nutrition from Bray GA, Popkin BM. Dietary fat intake does affect obesity! *Am J Clin Nutr* 1998;68: 1156–73, ©American Journal of Clinical Nutrition/American Society for Clinical Nutrition

a

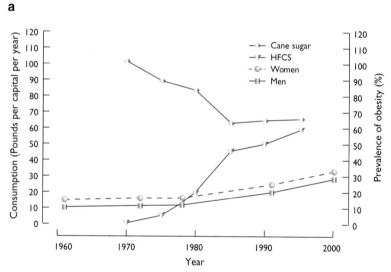

b

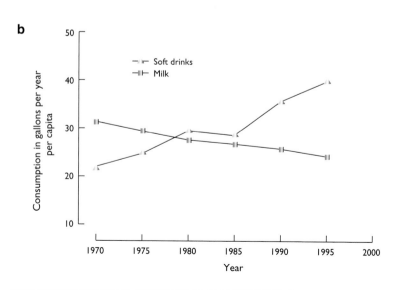

Figure 2.11 (a) High fructose corn sweeteners first entered the food supply in 1968 and after 1970 their consumption began to increase rapidly to the point where they represented nearly 50% of the sweeteners used by 1985 in the United States. This rise overlaps with the rate of increase in the prevalence of obesity. (b) The use of high corn products as sweeteners in regular soft drinks increases 'sweetness' because fructose is sweeter than sucrose and may play an important role in the increased consumption of soft drinks. Over the same interval that the consumption of regular soft drinks has increased, that of milk has decreased thus reducing the population's intake of calcium. HFCS, high fructose corn sweetener. Data derived from US Food Consumption 1970–97 by the United States Department of Agriculture

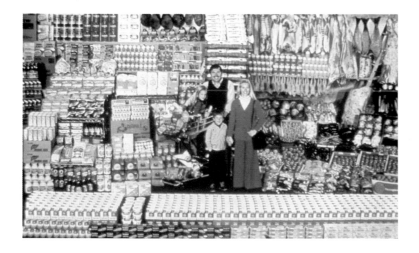

Figure 2.12 Food for a family of four for one year. Courtesy of Dr. Judith Stem

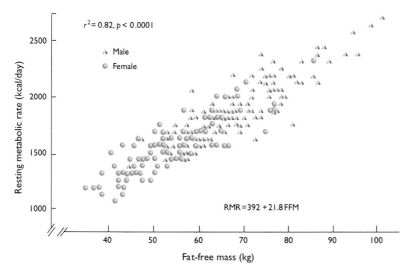

Figure 2.13 In human beings, energy expenditure measured in the metabolic chamber is best represented by the fat-free body mass. RMR, resting metabolic rate; FFM, fat-free mass. Adapted with permission from Ravussin E, Lillioja S, Anderson TE, Bogardus C. Determinants of 24-hour energy expenditure in man. Methods and results using a respiratory chamber. *J Clin Invest* 1986; 78:1568–78

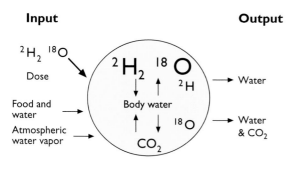

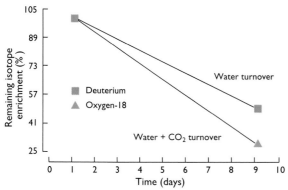

Figure 2.14 Energy expenditure can be measured by administering double-labled water($^2H^{18}O$). Since the hydrogen can be eliminated only as water in the urine, whereas the oxygen can be eliminated as both water and CO_2, the ratio of these two isotopes diverges and the rate of this divergence is a measure of CO_2 production. With an estimate of CO_2 production, it is then possible to calculate oxygen uptake. The model shown demonstrates this sequence

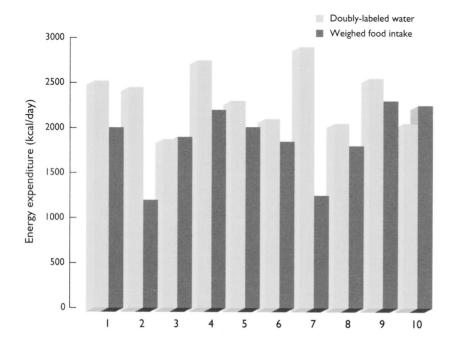

Figure 2.15 Diagram showing the average energy expenditure for 10 individual women determined by doubly-labeled water (left hand bar of each set) and the corresponding estimate of energy expenditure using a weighed food record (right hand bar of each set) obtained during the same 7 days that energy expenditure was measured. Note that in all but two the estimated energy from food intake is less than measured by doubly-labeled water, indicating that food records consistently underperform relative to doubly-labeled water. Adapted with permission from Champagne CM, Bray GA, Kurtz AA, et al. Energy intake and energy expenditure: a controlled study comparing dietitians and non-dietitians. J Am Diet Assoc 2002;102:1428–32

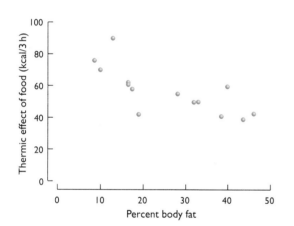

Figure 2.16 Thermic effect of food. A hooded canopy can be used to measure both resting metabolic rate and the thermic response to a meal. In studies of carefully matched individuals, there is a clear reduction in the thermic effect of a meal in obese individuals that appears to be related to the degree of insulin resistance in these individuals. Data derived from Segal KR, Albu J, Chun A, et al. Independent effects of obesity and insulin resistance on postprandial thermogenesis in men. J Clin Invest 1992;89:824–33

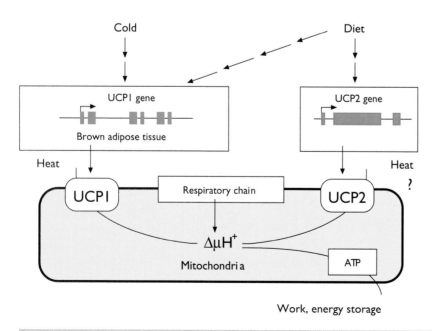

Figure 2.17 Uncoupling proteins. A family of uncoupling proteins has been identified in humam beings and in animals. Uncoupling protein (UCP)-1 is involved in dissipating energy, and is primarily located in the mitochondria of brown adipose tissue. UCP2 is widely distributed and appears to be involved in the transport of fatty acids across the mitochondrion. UCP3 is found primarily in muscle and may have a similar function to UCP2. Adapted with permission from Fleury C, Neverova M, Collins S, et al. Uncoupling protein-2: a noval gene linked to obesity and hyper-insulinemia. Nat Genet 1997;15:269–72

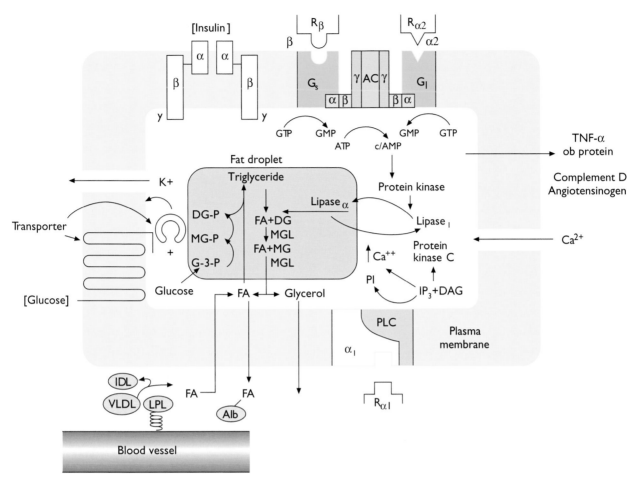

Figure 2.18   The fat cell is a complex hormonally regulated cell

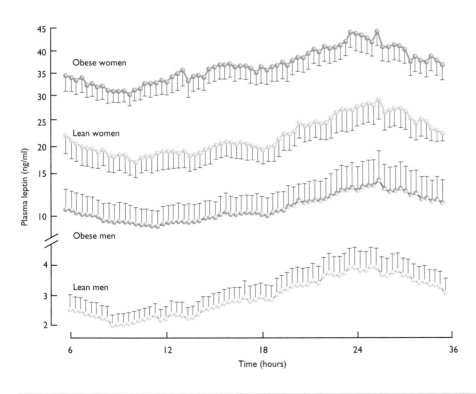

Figure 2.19 Leptin is probably the most important circulating peptide produced by the fat cell. When it is deficient in either humans or animals, obesity is one result. Its levels are normally higher in women than in men, and in obese subjects compared to lean subjects. There is a clear diurnal variation with the highest levels between 10.00 pm and 3.00 am. Data derived from Saad MF, Riad-Gabriel MG, Khan A, *et al.* Diurnal and ultradian rhythmicity of plasma leptin: effects of gender and adiposity. *J Clin Endocrinol Metab* 1998;83:453–9

1.	Leptin is synthesized in fat cells and placenta
2.	Women have higher leptin levels than men
3.	More fat means more leptin
4.	Leptin acts in the brain ovary liver hematopoietic cells
5.	Leptin deficiency produces obesity
6.	Leptin modifies effect of starvation
7.	Leptin is secreted in mother's milk
8.	Leptin is inversely related to menarcheal age
9.	Cord-blood leptin is related to birth weight
10.	Low leptin may predict weight gain
11.	Leptin increased in choriocarcinoma and hydatidiform mole

Figure 2.20 All you ever wanted to know about leptin but were afraid to ask

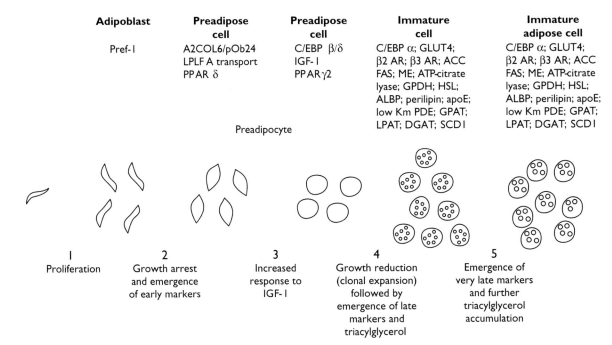

Figure 2.21 Development of the white fat cell. Pref-1, preadipocyte factor-1; A2COL6/pOb 24 = C/EBP β/δ = CCAAT/enhancer binding proteins β or δ; IGF-1, insulin-like growth hormone-1; PPARγ2, peroxisome proliferator-activated receptor γ-2; GLUT-4, glucose transporter-4; β2 AR, β-2 adrenergic receptor; β3 AR, β-3 adrenergic receptor; ACC, acetyl CoA carboxylase; FAS, fatty acid synthase; ME, malic enzyme, ATP: citrate lyase, adenosine triphosphate lyase; GPDH, glycerol 3-phosphate dehydrogenase; HSL, hormone sensitive lipase; ALBP, adipocyte fatty acid binding protein; low Km PDE, low Km phosphodiesterase; GPAT, glycerol phosphate acetyl transferase; LPAT, lyso-phosphoacyl transferase; DGAT, diglycerol acyltransferase, SCD1, stearoyl-coenzyme A desaturase

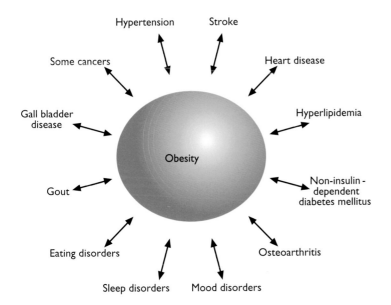

Figure 3.1 Conditions associated with obesity. The relationship of obesity to a variety of risks is shown in this diagram. Some of these risk factors can be related directly to the mass of extra fat (joint disease, sleep apnea, psychological responses) whereas others reflect metabolic consequences of an enlarged fat organ (diabetes, hypertension, heart disease, gall bladder disease and some forms of cancer)

Disease	Direct cost (billions)
Diabetes mellitus	$32.4
Coronary heart disease	$ 7.0
Osteoarthritis	$ 4.3
Hypertension	$ 3.2
Gallbladder disease	$ 2.6
Colon cancer	$ 1.0
Breast cancer	$ 0.84
Endometrial cancer	$ 0.29
	$51.63

Figure 3.2 Costs associated with obesity. This table shows an estimate of the direct costs of obesity in the United States in 1995. In addition to contributing to 300 000 extra deaths each year, there are large costs associated with the care of diseases attributed to obesity. Such estimates now exist in a number of countries and range from 2–7% of gross domestic product. Data derived from Wolf AM, Colditz GA. Current estimates of the economic costs of obesity in the United States. *Obes Res* 1998;6:97–106

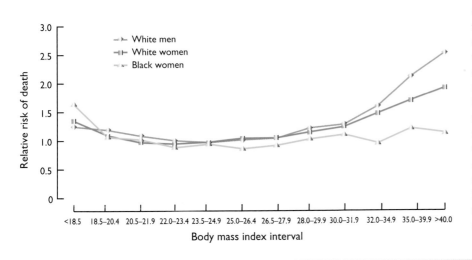

Figure 3.3 A higher body weight or body mass index (BMI) increases the risk of death. The overall risk of obesity has a curvilinear relationship to BMI {Wt(kg)/[Ht(m)]^2} used to express the rising body weight. This data is derived from the American Cancer Society Study II. This relationship is most evident in men and to a somewhat lesser extent in women and even less in African-American (black) women. Data derived from Calle EE, Thun MJ, Petrelli JM, *et al.* Body-mass index and mortality in a prospective cohort of U.S. adults. *N Engl J Med* 1999;341:1097–105

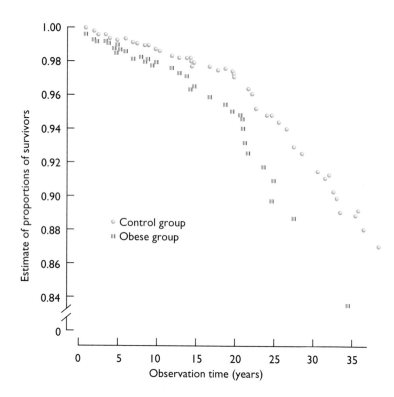

Figure 3.4 The detrimental effect of obesity on longevity continues over many years. These data show the proportion of men surviving over years after their evaluation for service in the Danish military, depending on whether they were obese or not. The group of obese men (BMI > 31 kg/m²) had fewer survivors at all times up to 35 years following initial evaluation. Adapted with permission from Sonne-Holm S, Sorensen TI, Christensen U. Risk of early death in extremely overweight young men. *Br Med J* 1983;287:795–7

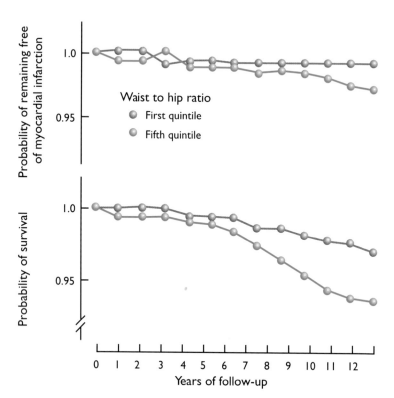

Figure 3.5 An increase in central fat also increases the risk of mortality and of several diseases. This is shown using data from this Swedish study. The central fat was estimated from the ratio of the wasit circumference divided by the hip circumference (WHR) in men. Over the 12 years of the study, the individuals in the top twentieth percentile for WHR had a shorter life expectancy than the women in the lowest twentieth percentile. Adapted with permission from Lapidus L, Bengtsson C, Larsson B, *et al.* Distribution of adipose tissue and risk of cardiovascular death: a 12 year follow up of participants in the population study of women in Gothenburg, Sweden. *Br Med J* 1984;289:1257–61

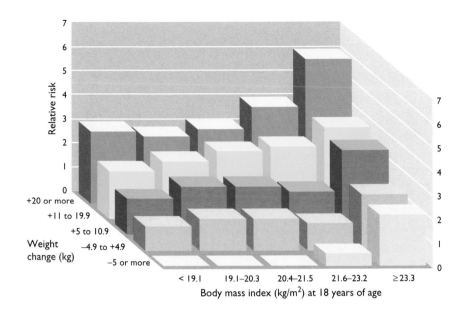

Figure 3.6 Weight gain in both men and women after the age of 18–20 years is associated with increased mortality and with an increase in the risk of several diseases. This figure from the Nurses' Health Study shows, as does Figure 3.3 that relative risk increases in individuals with higher body mass index (BMI). It also shows that the more weight these women gained the greater the risk at any given BMI. Adapted with permission from Willett WC, Manson JE, Stampfer MJ, et al. Weight, weight change and coronary heart disease in women. Risk within the 'normal' weight range. J Am Med Assoc 1995;273:461–5,©1995 American Medical Association

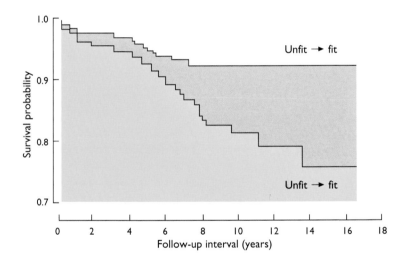

Figure 3.7 Physical fitness also impacts on the health risks of an individual. Those that were initially physically unfit and then improved their fitness through regular physical activity had a better likelihood of survival than individuals who remained unfit over the 17 years of follow-up. Data derived from Blair SN, Kohn HW 3rd, Paffenbarger RS Jr, et al. Physical fitness and all-cause mortality. A prospective study of healthy men and women. J Am Med Assoc 1989; 262: 2395–2401

Age adjusted odds ratio for BMI > 40 kg/m²						
	Men			**Women**		
Disease	**White**	**African American**	**Mexican American**	**White**	**African American**	**Mexican American**
Diabetes (NIDDM)	24.3	5.1	12.2	15.7	20.0	4.6
Hypertension	6.8	14.4	22.5	10.4	3.5	3.1
Gallbladder disease	12.5	—	6.5	7.8	9.8	4.4
Coronary heart disease	2.6	1.5	7.0	3.3	2.8	5.4
High cholesterol	2.3	1.5	0.8	1.1	1.7	0.8

Figure 3.8 The risks for many diseases differ by ethnic groups. This is shown in this table using data for individuals with a body mass index > 40 kg/m². For example, the highest risk of diabetes was in white men and African-American women. Hypertension, on the other hand, had a higher likelihood of developing in the Mexican-American men and the white women. Data derived from Must A, Spadano J, Coakley EH, et al. The disease burden associated with overweight and obesity. J Am Med Assoc 1999;282:1523–9

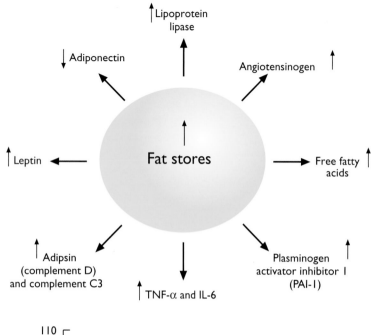

Figure 3.9 The fat cell is an endocrine cell, and part of an endocrine organ that is widely dispersed. The cell produces a variety of peptides and several metabolites. The pathological lesion in obesity is hypertrophy or enlargement of these fat cells. The enhanced secretion of peptides and metabolites from fat cells contributes to the pathophysiologic processes resulting from obesity. Particularly important are the free fatty acids (FFA), notably when the latter are released into the portal vein and modify hepatic function, and the reduced levels of adiponectin

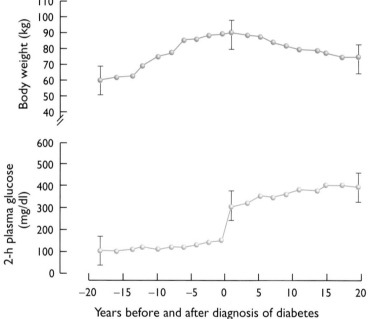

Figure 3.10 Weight gain precedes the onset of diabetes. These data from the Pima Indians show that there is a slow steady weight gain over the 10 years preceding the onset of diabetes, but that after that body weight begins to decline slowly. Adapted with permission of The American Diabetes Association from Ravussin E. Energy metabolism in obesity. Studies in the Pima Indians. *Diabetes Care* 1993;16:232–8, ©1993 American Diabetes Association

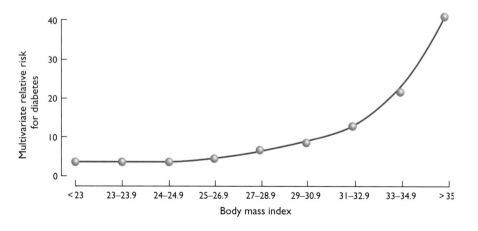

Figure 3.11 A higher body mass index (BMI) is associated with a higher risk of diabetes. When the BMI exceeds 35 kg/m², this risk increases to more than 20-fold above those with a BMI below 23 kg/m². A loss of body weight reduces the risk of developing diabetes significantly. Data derived from Colditz FA, Willett WC, Rotnitzky A, Manson JE. Weight gain as a risk factor for clinical diabetes mellitus in women. *Ann Intern Med* 1995;122:481–6

Waist (cm)	< 88	88–91	92–96	96–102	> 102
Relative risk of NIDDM*	1.0	1.2	1.5	1.7	3.1

*Adjusted for age, family history, smoking, BMI

Figure 3.12 Central obesity increases the risk of diabetes. There was a graded increase in the risk of diabetes for men as their waist circumference, an index of central adiposity, increased. Data derived from Chan JM, Rimm EB, Colditz GA, *et al.* Obesity, fat distribution, and weight gain as risk factors for clinical diabetes in men. *Diabetes Care* 1994;17:961–9

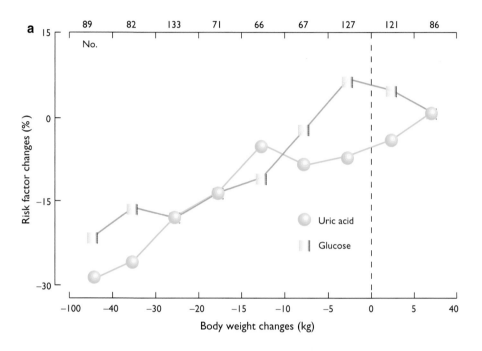

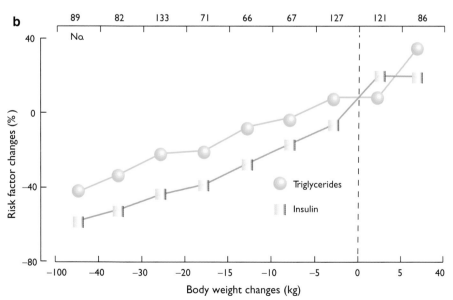

Figure 3.13 Weight loss improves the metabolic variables associated with diabetes. In data from the Swedish Obese Subjects Study there was a graded reduction in glucose, uric acid (a), insulin and triglycerides (b) with increasing degrees of weight loss. Adapted with permission from Sjostrom CD, Lissner L, Sjostrom L. Relationship between changes in body composition and changes in cardiovascular risk factors: the SOS Intervention Study. Swedish Obese Subjects. *Obes Res* 1997;5:519–30

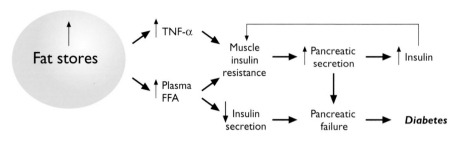

Figure 3.14 A pathophysiological model can relate the changes in fatty acid secretion to the altered responses that lead to diabetes and insulin resistance. Insulin resistance is an important part of the metabolic syndrome which also includes central adiposity, low HDL-cholesterol, high triglycerides and hypertension

Syndrome	Clinical features	Mechanisms
Type A syndrome		
Classic	Acanthosis nigricans, severe insulin resistance, ovarian hyperandrogenism	Insulin-receptor mutations or other target-cell defects in insulin action
Rabson-Mendenhall	Type A features, perhaps with dental dysplasia, pineal hyperplasia, or other dysmorphic features	Insulin-receptor mutations or other target-cell defects in insulin action; possibly other defects
Pseudo-acromegaly	Type A features, perhaps with acral enlargement, muscle hypertrophy, widened teeth spacing, muscle cramps, or other features of acromegaly	Possibly insulin-receptor mutations, other defects
Leprechaunism	Intrauterine growth retardation dysmorphic facies, perhaps with Type A features, hypertrichosis, lipoatrophy, or phallic enlargement	Insulin-receptor mutations; possible defects in other growth-factor receptors or pathways common to multiple growth factors
Lipodystrophy Total congenital lipoatrophy	Total lipoatrophy, perhaps with Type A features, hepatosplenomegaly, cardiomyopathy, features of acromegaly, hypertriglyceridemia, or genital hypertrophy	Possibly insulin-receptor mutations or other defects
Partial congenital lipodystrophy	Adipose-tissue depots variably affected by lipoatrophy or lipohypertrophy perhaps with Type A features, hepatosplenomegaly, cardiomyopathy, features of acromegaly, hypertriglyceridemia	Possibly insulin-receptor mutations or other defects

Figure 3.15 Syndromes of insulin resistance. In addition to the relation of insulin resistance to central adiposity, there are a number of clinical syndromes that have insulin resistance as a prominent feature. The genetic forms of syndromes of insulin resistance are summarized in the table

Effects of a 9 kg weight loss		Reduced risk
Cholesterol	↓ 10 mg/dl	↓ 10%
HDL-cholesterol	↑ 3 mg/dl	↓ 6%
Blood pressure	↓ 5 mmHg	↓ 15%
		31%

Figure 3.16 Obesity and risk for cardiovascular disease. For each 9 kg change in weight there are significant changes in cholesterol, HDL-cholesterol and blood pressure that contribute to the risk of obesity for developing heart disease. Data derived from Gundy SM. Overview: The role of diet in the prevention of heart disease. In Bray GA, Ryan DH, eds. *Nutrition, Genetics and Heart Disease.* Pennington Center Nutrition Series, Vol. 6. Baton Rouge, LA: Louisiana State University Press, 1996:1–11

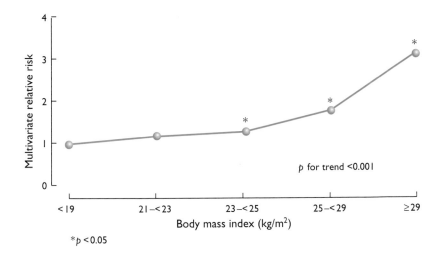

p for trend <0.001

*p <0.05

Figure 3.17 The body mass index is related to the risk of heart disease. Data derived from Manson JE, Willett WC, Stampfer MJ, *et al.* Body weight and mortality among women. *N Engl J Med* 1995;333:677–85

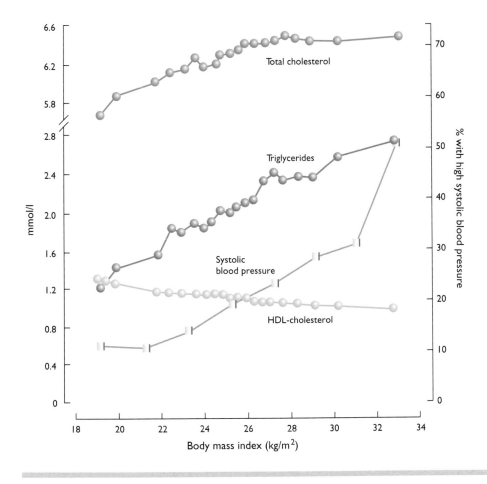

Figure 3.18 Body mass index is also related to higher levels of total cholesterol, triglycerides and systolic blood pressure and to a decreased level of HDL-cholesterol which are risk factors for disease. Adapted with permission from Pocock SJ, Shaper AG, Phillips AN. Concentrations of high-density lipoprotein cholesterol, triglycerides and total cholesterol in ischaemic heart disease. Data derived from Shaper AG, Phillips AN, Pocock SJ, *et al.* Risk factors for stroke in middle aged British men. *Br Med J* 1991; 302; 1111-5.

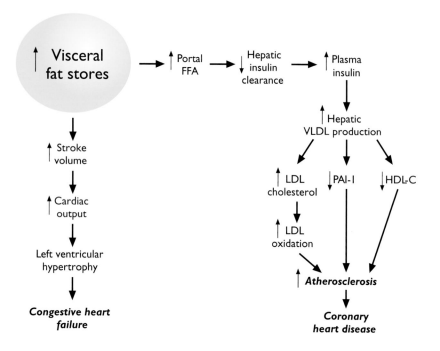

Figure 3.19 This figure shows a pathophysiological model of how the changes in these risk factors might develop as a result of increased levels of free fatty acids (FFA). FFA released into the portal vein may reduce insulin clearance by the liver and enhance triglyceride production while reducing HDL-cholesterol (HDL-C) levels. This set of events along with the higher levels of plasminogen activator inhibitor-1 (PAI-1) produced by the enlarged fat cells increases the risk of atherosclerosis

Variable	Non-obese (n = 25)	Obese: level of deep abdominal fat	
		Low (n = 10)	High (n = 10)
% Body fat	28.0 ± 5.6	47.0 ± 6.4	49.8 ± 3.2
Deep abdominal fat area (cm²)	50.3 ± 16.8	107.0 ± 33.4	186.7 ± 36.8
Triglyceride (mmol/l)	0.79 ± 0.35	1.47 ± 0.79	2.57 ± 2.41
Cholesterol (mmol/l)	4.59 ± 0.88	5.18 ± 0.93	5.65 ± 1.23
LDL-cholesterol (mmol/l)	3.0 ± 0.87	3.56 ± 0.92	3.81 ± 1.10
HDL-cholesterol (mmol/l)	1.36 ± 0.24	1.25 ± 0.18	0.96 ± 0.12
Fasting insulin (pmol/l)	39.0 ± 12.4	91.5 ± 59.9	150.3 ± 57.3
Glucose area ([mmol/l/180 min] × 10^{-3})	10.7 ± 0.19	1.14 ± 0.22	1.40 ± 0.19
Insulin area ([pmol/l/180 min] × 10^{-3})	46.6 ± 19.4	82.1 ± 48.3	121.0 ± 39.5

Figure 3.20 Visceral or central obesity, here measured by CT scans, is related to abnormal levels of lipids. Clinically, the waist circumference and the sagittal diameter appear to estimate the lipid abnormalities in men and women better than the waist-to-hip ratio and is now used in epidemiological studies. Data derived from Despres JP, Moorjani S, Lupien PJ, et al. Regional distribution of body fat, plasma lipoproteins, and cardiovascular disease. *Arteriosclerosis* 1990;10:497–511

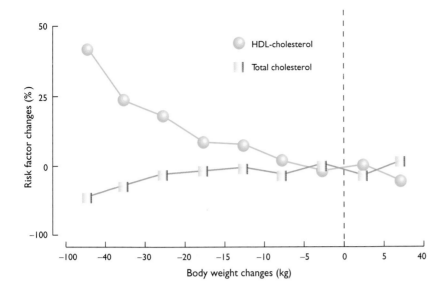

Figure 3.21 Weight loss reduces total cholesterol and raises HDL-cholesterol. It is particularly note-worthy that the reduction in total cholesterol does not occur until the weight loss reaches 20-30 kg, compared to the graded increase in HDL-cholesterol with each increment in weight loss. Adapted with permission from Sjostrom CD, Lissner L, Sjostrom L. Relationships between changes in body composition and changes in cardiovascular risk factors: the SOS Intervention Study. *Obes Res* 1997;5:519–30

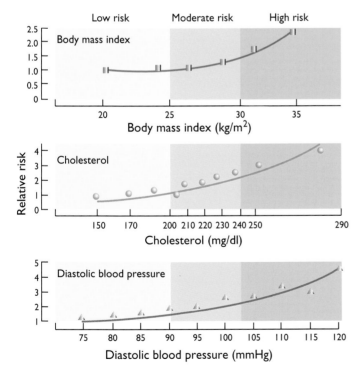

Figure 3.22 Body mass index, cholesterol and diastolic blood pressure each show a similar curvilinear relation with mortality rates. Courtesy of George A. Bray

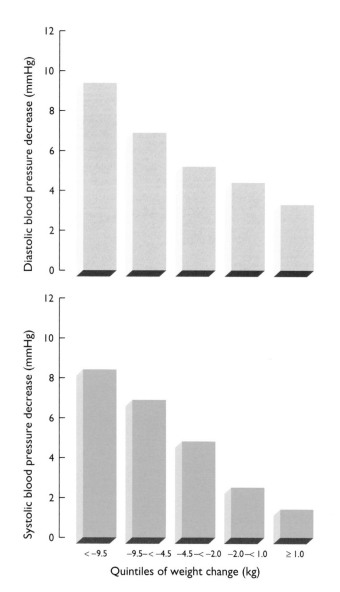

Figure 3.23 Weight loss reduces blood pressure over the first 2–4 years, but with longer maintenance of weight loss there is a recovery of blood pressure to normal levels. Data derived from Stevens VJ, Codrrigan SA, Obarzanek E, *et al.* Weight loss intervention in phase 1 of the Trials of Hypertension Prevention. The TOHP Collaborative Research Group. *Arch Intern Med* 1993;153:849–58

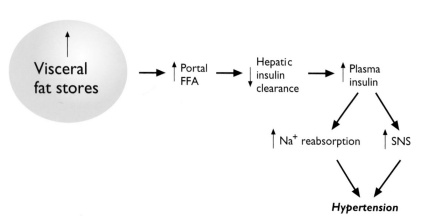

Figure 3.24 A pathophysiological model for the risk of developing hypertension. SNS, sympathetic nervous system

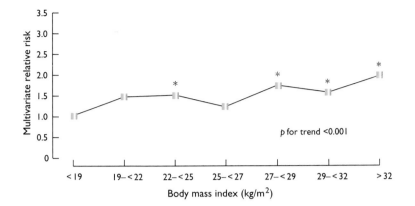

Figure 3.25 The relationship of body mass index to the risk of cancer. There is an increase in selected cancers, namely in the uterus, ovary, breast, gall bladder, colon and prostate with increasing weight that is most noticeable when the BMI is above 30 kg/m². Data derived from Manson JE, Willett WC, Stampfer MJ, *et al.* Body weight and mortality among women. *N Engl J Med* 1995;333:677–85

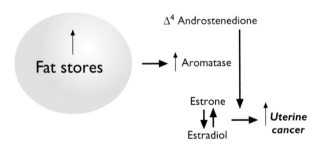

Figure 3.26 A pathophysiological model for risk of breast and uterine cancer in obese post-menopausal women. When estrogen production by the ovary fails, the major source is the conversion of androstenedione to estrone in adipose tissue. Obese women having larger fat deposits convert larger amounts of this precursor to estrone and thus enhance the estrogenic effects on breast and uterus

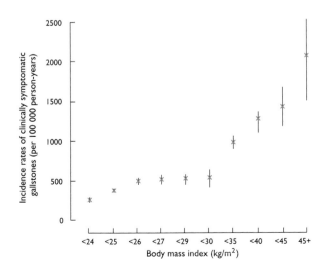

Figure 3.27 The relation of the increasing body mass index to the risk for gall bladder disease. Adapted with permission of the American Journal of Clinical Nutrition from Stampfer MJ, Maclure KM, Colditz GA, *et al.* Risk of symptomatic gallstones in women with severe obesity. *Am J Clin Nutr* 1992;55:652–8, © American Journal of Clinical Nutrition/American Society for Clinical Nutrition

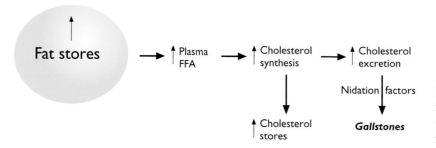

Figure 3.28 A pathophysiological model for the metabolism of cholesterol in the development of gall bladder disease. FFA, free fatty acids

1. Increased cortisol production

2. Insulin resistance

3. Decreased sex hormone binding globulin (SHBG) in women

4. Decreased progesterone levels in women

5. Decreased testosterone levels in men

6. Decreased growth hormone production

7. Increased 11-β-hydroxy steroid dehydrodenase levels

Figure 3.29 A number of endocrine complications have been associated with obesity. Data derived from World Health Organization. *Preventing and Managing the Global Epidemic.* Report of a WHO Consultation. Geneva: World Health Organization, Technical Report Series no. 894, 2000

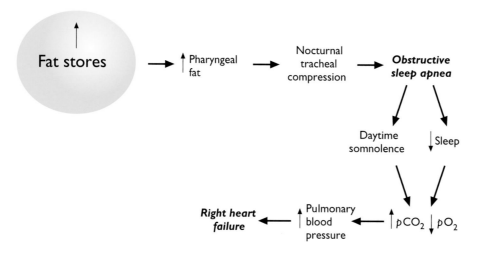

Figure 3.30 Sleep apnea is a common problem particularly in overweight men. One component of the problem is compression of the upper airway due to increased amounts of pharyngeal fat. The apneic periods produce difficulty sleeping at night and a tendency to somnolence during the day. If allowed to continue untreated, pulmonary hypertension and right heart failure can supervene

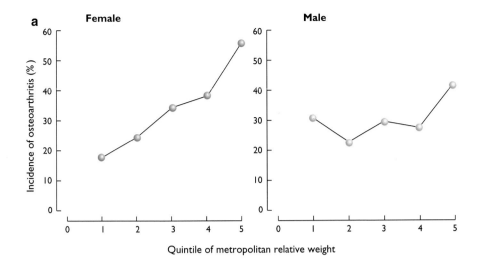

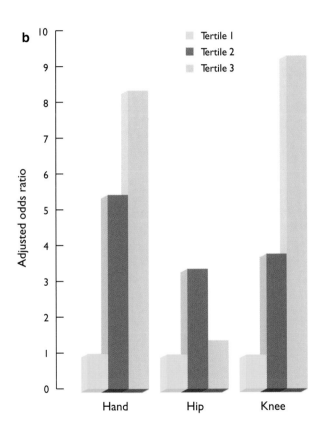

Figure 3.31 (a) The relationship of body mass index to the risk of developing osteoarthritis. Data derived from Felson DT, Anderson JJ, Naimark A, *et al.* Obesity and knee osteoarthritis. The Framingham Study. *Ann Intern Med* 1988;109:18–24. (b) The odds ratio for the incidence of osteoarthritis in the hand, hip and knee using data from a case–control study of 134 women and matched controls whose arthritis began between 1990 and 1993. Adapted with permission from Oliveria SA, Felson DT, Cirilo PA, *et al.* Body weight, body mass index, and incident symptomatic osteoarthritis of the hand, hip, and knee. *Epidemiology* 1999;10:161–6

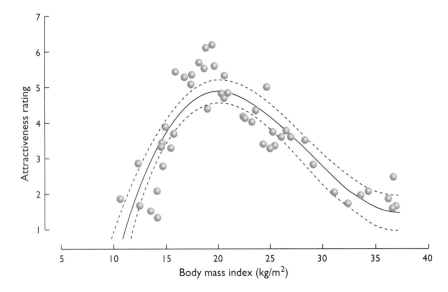

Figure 3.32 Obesity is a stigmatized condition. This is clear from the large preponderance of women seeking help to lose weight. It is also shown in this figure relating an attractiveness rating to body mass index. Adapted with permission of Elsevier Science from Tovée MJ, Reinhardt S, Emery JL, Cornelissen PL. Optimum body-mass index and maximum sexual attractiveness. *Lancet* 1998;352:548

Variable	Observed value		
	Overweight (n = 195)	Non-overweight (n = 4943)	p value
Married (%) (n = 4922)	28%	56%	< 0.001
Household income ($) (n = 4286)	$18 372	$30 586	< 0.001
Income below poverty level (%)† (n = 4286)	32%	13%	< 0.001
Education (year) (n = 4881)	12.1	13.1	0.009
Completed college (%) (n = 4881)	9%	21%	0.21
Self-esteem in 1987 (n = 5138)	32.4	33.6	0.38
†Household poverty was defined according to federal poverty guidelines			

Figure 3.33 The effects of obesity on psychosocial difficulties. Overweight adolescent women were less likely to marry, had lower incomes and less education. Adapted with permission from Gortmaker SL, Must A, Perin JM, *et al*. Social and economic consequences of overweight in adolescence and young adulthood. *N Engl J Med* 1993; 329: 1008–12, ©1993 Massachusetts Medical Society. All rights reserved

Sleep apnea
Blount's disease
Slipped capital femoral epiphysis
NIDDM
Polycystic ovary syndrome
Hypertension
Dyslipidemias

Figure 3.34 Complications of childhood obesity. The most striking consequence of increasing obesity in children has been the appearance of obesity in adolescents from Latino or African-American ancestry associated with a distressing increase in the rate of type 2 diabetes (NIDDM, non-insulin-dependent diabetes mellitus)

Anatomic characteristics
Total body fat
Regional fat distribution
Visceral fat/metabolic syndrome
Lipomas and abnormal fat deposits

Etiologic classification
Hypothalamic
Endocrine
Dietary
Physical inactivity
Drug -induced
Genetic

Functional classification
Insulin resistance/metabolic syndrome
Hypertension
Gall bladder dysfunction
Cardiomyopathy
Sleep apnea
Depression
Restraint/binge eating
Osteoarthritis

Associated risks
High blood pressure (systolic >140 mmHg, diastolic > 90 mmHg)
Diabetes (>126 mg/dl) or fasting hyperglycemia (110–126 mg/dl)
Hyperinsulinemia (>15 μU/ml) or insulin resistance
Total cholesterol ÷ HDL cholesterol (females > 5.0, males > 6.0)
LVH by ECG
Sleep apnea or high $PaCO_2$
Hirsutism or high LH/FSH ratio

Figure 4.1 A classification of obesity. Four different classifications are included in this table. The first is an anatomic classification based on the size, number, location and histological characteristics of fat cells. Since the sine qua non of obesity is an enlargement of the fat cell, consideration of the anatomic features of this problem provides a useful way to classify it. The second classification is based on the definable causes or etiologies of obesity. For the clinician it is important to identify those types of obesity that can be separated off based on phenotypic features, from the larger group of obesities where the only obvious phenotype is increased fatness. The third classification is functional and based on the disease entities associated with obesity. The final classification is whether or not patients have the metabolic syndrome or other associated conditions

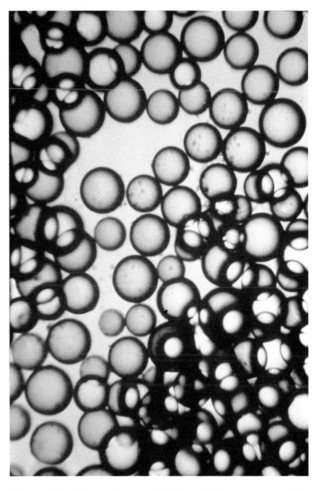

Figure 4.2 Photomicrograph of fat cells from an overweight individual following trypsin digestion. The variation in size is evident but when compared to similar preparations from normal weight individuals, the average cell size is clearly enlarged

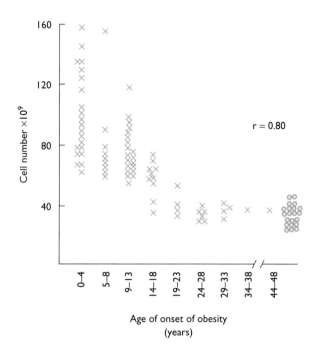

r = 0.80

Figure 4.3 A second characteristic of the fat mass is the number of fat cells. The control of fat cell differentiation and multiplication is a complex process. The adipoblast in the presence of insulin, cortisol and others factors begins the process of differentiation to the preadipocyte. During this transition the protein pattern of the cell changes as the genes controlling differentiation are activated. For the differentiation from a preadipocyte into a mature adipocyte peroxisome proliferator-activated receptors (PPAR- α and γ) play a key role. The thiazolidinedione class of drugs activates these receptors and enhances the rate of development for small fat cells. This figure shows the number of fat cells in individuals of various ages using fat biopsies from three different adipose deposits to estimate fat cell size and an estimate of the total fat from isotope dilution. Note that individuals who become obese as youngsters often have markedly increased numbers of fat cells. Individuals who become markedly obese as adults may also increase their number of fat cells. Reproduced with permission from Salans LB, Cushman SW, Weisman RE. Adipose cell size and number in nonobese and obese patients. *J Clin Invest* 1973;52:929–41

Causes of hypothalamic obesity
Hypothalamic lesion
1. Tumors
2. Inflammation
3. Trauma
Endocrine disturbances
1. Amenorrhea/impotence
2. Impaired growth
3. Diabetes insipidus
4. Thyroid/adrenal insufficiency
Intracranial pressure
1. Papilledema
2. Vomiting
Neurological disturbances
1. Thirst
2. Somnolence

Figure 4.4 Several kinds of hypothalamic disease can cause human obesity. The basic causes are shown in this table

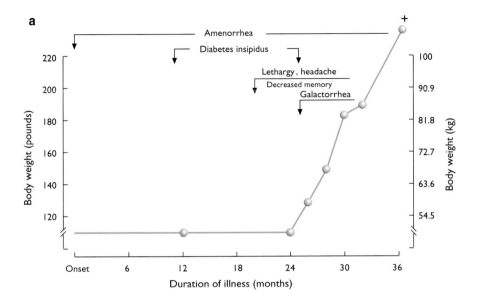

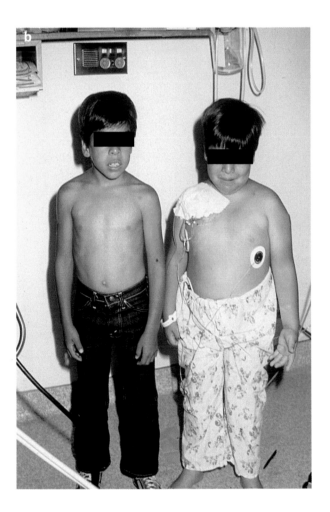

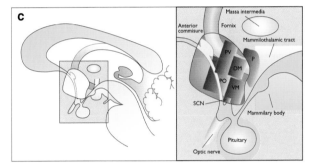

Figure 4.5 (a) This figure shows the clinical course of one patient with hypothalamic obesity due to tuberculomas. After developing a number of endocrine symptoms, she gained 50 kg in her last year. (b) This pictures shows identical twins aged 11. The twin on the right had a sudden episode of convulsions that was probably caused by hypernatremia. His subsequent endocrine history reveals a number of transient changes with eventual onset of obesity and short stature that is probably the result of an injury to the hypothalamus. He is shorter and heavier than his brother and had small shoe and hand size. (c) This picture is one of the few autopsies that have carefully examined the hypothalamus of a patient who died from hypothalamic obesity. The area that was damaged includes the paraventricular nucleus and the ventromedial hypothalamus. Adapted with permission from Haugh RM, Markesbery WR. Hypothalamic astrocytoma. Syndrome of hyperphagia, obesity and disturbances of behavior and endocrine and autonomic function. *Arch Neurol* 1983;40: 560–3

a	Cushing's syndrome
	• Central obesity
	• Hypertension
	• Plethoric facies
	• Amenorrhea
	• Virilism
	• Edema of lower extremities
	• Hemorrhagic features

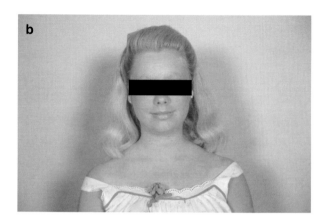

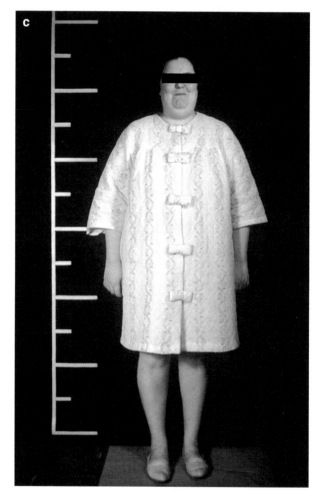

Figure 4.6 (a) Cushing's syndrome resulting from a basophilic adenoma of the pituitary gland was originally described by Harvey Cushing in 1932. One clinical feature of these patients is weight gain with most of the weight being centrally located. Hypertension and abdominal striae are also common. Increased cortisol secretion is the main cause of the problem. When this occurs in children not only do they become obese, but linear growth ceases. (b) Picture of an adolescent with Cushing's syndrome whose symptoms were weight gain, cessation of menses, a round plethoric face and linear growth. (c) A grown woman with increased blood pressure, amenorrhea, abdominal and cervical fatness

Polycystic ovary syndrome

- Oligomenorrhea/amenorrhea
- Hirsutism
- Polycystic ovaries
- ↑LH/FSH
- ↑Testosterone/↓SHBG
- Insulin resistance
- Normal IGF-I
- ↓IGF-I binding protein

Figure 4.7 The polycystic ovary syndrome is another endocrine disease in which obesity commonly manifests itself. The features of this syndrome are shown in this table. Ultrasound of the ovary can show the polycystic nature of this organ

Category	Drugs which cause weight gain	Possible alternatives
Neuroleptics	Thioridazine; olanzepine; quetiapine; resperidone	Molindone; haldol; ziprasodone

Antidepressants
  Tricyclics
  Monoamine oxidase inhbitors
  Selective serotonin reuptake inhibitors
	Amitriptyline;
	Imipramine
	Paroxetine
		Protriptyline; bupropion; nefazodone; fluoxetine; sertraline

Anticonvulsants	Valproate; carbamazepine; gabapentin	Topiramate; lamotrigine
Antidiabetic drugs	Insulin Sulfonylureas Thiazolidinediones	Inhaled insulin Miglitol; acarbose Metformin
β-Adrenergic blockers	Propranolol	ACE Inhibitors; calcium channel blockers
Steroid hormones	Contraceptives Glucocorticoids Progestational steroids	Barrier methods Non-steroidal anti-inflammatory agents

Figure 4.8 As the number of receptor-specific medications has increased, several classes of them have been associated with weight gain. This table lists the more common groups. The drugs used to treat psychiatric diseases, particularly the more recent atypical dopamine antagonists, are particularly problematic. Most anti-diabetic drugs, including insulin, sulfonylureas and thiazolidinediones, are also associated with weight gain.

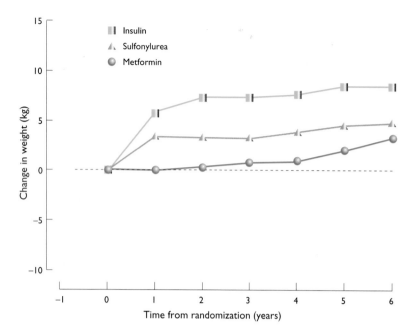

Figure 4.9 The weight gain reported in patients treated with sulfonylureas and insulin compared to the smaller gain with metformin in the United Kingdom Prospective Diabetes Study is shown here. Over the course of the trial the metformin group was similar to the controls, but the other two gained significant amounts of weight. Adapted with permission of Elsevier Science from UK Prospective Diabetes Study (UKPDS) Group. Effect of intensive blood-glucose control with metformin on complications in overweight patients with type 2 diabetes (UKPDS 34). *Lancet* 1998;352: 854–65

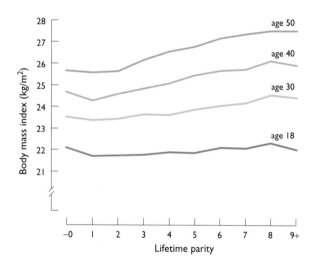

Figure 4.10 Pregnancy is associated with weight gain. This is particularly true for women with more than one pregnancy. This effect on BMI is shown here. Adapted with permission from Brown JE, Kaye SA, Folsom AR. Parity-related weight change in women. *Int J Obes Relat Metab Dis* 1992;16:627–31

a

Gene	Mutations	Chromosome	Number and sex	Age	Weight (kg)	BMI kg/m[2]	References
Pro-opiomelanocortin (POMC)	G701T and C deletion at nt 7133 exon 3 C3804A exon 2	2p23	1 F 1 M	3 7	30 50		Krude et al., 1998[1]
Melanocortin 4-receptor	C705A (Tyr 35X) ΔCTCT frame shift nt 631–634 codon 211 Y35X (also D37V) (S30F; P78L; T112M; R165W; G252S; I317T)	18q21.3	4 F 5 M	4 to 58		28–57	Vaisse C, et al., 2000[2]; Farooqi et al., 2000[3]; Hinney et al., 1999[4]
Leptin	Deletion at codon 133 C to T codon 105 Exon 3	7q31	4 F 2 M	2 to 34	29 to 130	32–56	Montague et al., 1997[5]; Strobel et al., 1998[6]; Ozata et al., 1999[7]
Leptin receptor	G to A exon 16	1p31	3 F	13 to 19	133 to 166	52–72	Clement et al., 1998[8]
Prohormone convertase-1	G483R A to C intron 5	5q15–q21	1 F	3	36		Jackson et al., 1997[9]
Peroxisome proliferator-activated receptor-γ	P115Q	3p25	1 F 3 M	32–74		38–47	Ristow et al., 1998[10]
Thyroid hormone receptor-β	C434Stop C to A exon 10	3p24.1–p22	1 F	15	46	26	Behr et al., 1997[11]

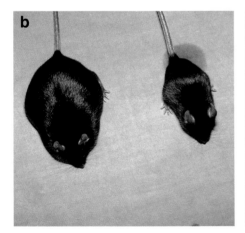

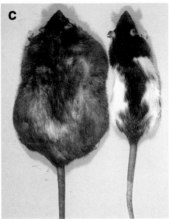

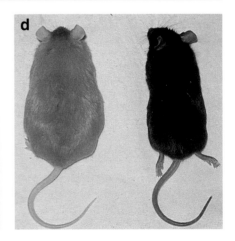

Figure 4.11 A variety of human syndromes of obesity that parallel syndromes described in animals have been reported. The features of these syndromes are summarized (a). In [1]Krude H, Biebermann H, Luck W, et al. Nat Genet 1998;19:155–7; [2]Vaisse C, Clement K, Durand E, et al. J Clin Invest 2000;106:253–62; [3]Farooqi IS, Yeo GS, Keogh JM, et al. J Clin Invest 2000;106:271–9; [4]Hinney A, Schmidt A, Nottlebom K, et al. I Clin Endocrinol Metab 1999;84:1483–6; [5]Montague CT, Farooqi IS, Whitehead JP, et al. Nature 1997;386:903–8; [6]Strobel A, Issad T, Camoin L, et al. Nat Genet 1998;18:213–5; [7]Ozata M, Ozdemir IC, Licinio J. J Clin Endocrinol 1999;84:3686–95; [8]Clement K, Vaisse C, Lahlou N, et al. Nature 1998;392:398–401; [9]Jackson RS, Creerners JW, Onagi S, et al. Nat Genet 1997;16:303–6; [10]Ristow M, Muller-Wieland D, Pfeiffer A, et al. N Engl J Med 1998;339:953–9; [11]Behr M, Ramsden DB, Loos U. J Clin Endocrinol Metab 1997;82:1081–7. (b), (c) and (d) show mouse or rat models representing some of the human obesities listed in (a). The obese (ob/ob) mouse lacks leptin and is similar to the three known families with very obese individuals (b). The fatty rat lacks the leptin receptor and individuals with this defect in one family are also very fat (c). The agouti derangement in the yellow mouse produces an effect similar to the changes in the melanocortin-4 receptor that is associated with many cases of human obesity (d)

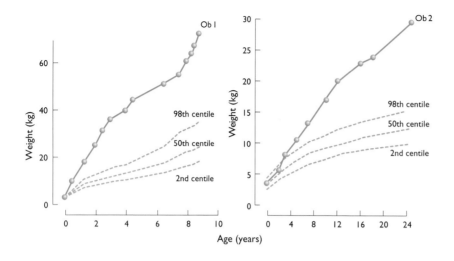

Figure 4.12 Weight gain in two children (*ob1 and ob2*) that are leptin-deficient. When these children were subsequently treated with leptin there was a significant loss in weight. Adapted with permission from Montague CT, Farooqi IS, Whitehead JP, *et al.* Congenital leptin deficiency is associated with severe early-onset obesity in humans. *Nature* 1997;387:903–8

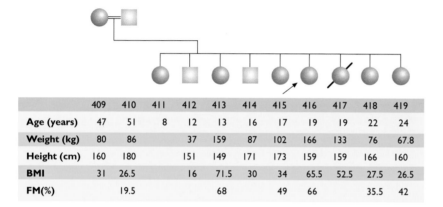

	409	410	411	412	413	414	415	416	417	418	419
Age (years)	47	51	8	12	13	16	17	19	19	22	24
Weight (kg)	80	86		37	159	87	102	166	133	76	67.8
Height (cm)	160	180		151	149	171	173	159	159	166	160
BMI	31	26.5		16	71.5	30	34	65.5	52.5	27.5	26.5
FM(%)		19.5			68		49	66		35.5	42

Figure 4.13 The family tree for leptin receptor deficiency. Only one such family has been reported, but they are resistant to treatment with leptin. FM, fat mass. Adapted with permission from Clement K, Vaisse C, Lahlou N, *et al.* A mutation in the human leptin receptor gene causes obesity and pituitary dysfunction. *Nature* 1998;392:398–401

	Syndrome				
Feature	**Prader–Willi**	**Bardet–Biedl**	**Ahlstrom**	**Cohen**	**Carpenter**
Inheritance	Sporadic 2/3 have defect	Autosomal-recessive	Autosomal-recessive	Probably autosomal-recessive	Autosomal-recessive
Stature	Short	Normal Infrequently short	Normal Infrequently short	Short or tall	Normal
Obesity	Generalized Moderate to severe onset 1–3 years	Generalized Early onset 1–2 years	Truncal Early onset 2–5 years	Truncal Mid childhood age 5	Truncal Gluteal mid-childhood
Cranofacies	Narrow bifrontal diameter Almond-shaped eyes Strabismus V-shaped mouth High arched palate	Not distinctive	Not distinctive	High nasal bridge Arched palate Open mouth Short philtrum	Acrocephaly Flat nasal bridge High arched palate
Limbs	Small hands and feet Hypotonia	Polydactyly	No abnormalities	Hypotonia Narrow hands and feet	Polydactyly Syndactyly Genu valgum
Reproductive status	Primary hypogonadism	Primary hypogonadism	Hypogonadism in males but not in females	Normal gonadal function or hypo-gonadotropic hypogonadism	Secondary hypogonadism
Other features	Enamel hypoplasia Hyperphagia Temper tantrums Nasal speech			Dysplastic ears Delayed puberty	
Mental retardation	Mild to moderate		normal IQ	Mild	Slight

Figure 4.14 Syndromic forms of obesity most of which include hypogonadism and mental retardation. This group of five syndromes include the Prader–Willi syndrome which is the most common one to be observed clinically

Clinical findings in Prader–Willi syndrome		
		%
Gestation	Poor fetal vigor	84
	Breech presentation	38
	Non-term delivery	33
Neonatal and infancy	Low birth weight (< 5 lb)	100
		90
	Delayed milestones	90
Central nervous system	Mental retardation	100
	Seizures	20
	Personality problems	71
Growth	Obesity	100
	Short stature	90
	Delayed bone age	90
Facies	Strabismus	95
Limbs	Small hands and feet	100
Sexual development	Cryptorchidism (males)	100
	Hypogenitalism (males)	100
	Menstruation	33

Figure 4.15 The Prader–Willi syndrome is probably the commonest phenotypic syndrome of obesity resulting from a deletion or translocation in chromosome 15. The gene loss has not yet been pinpointed. Clinically these individuals are a challenge. Help can be found from the Prader–Willi Foundation

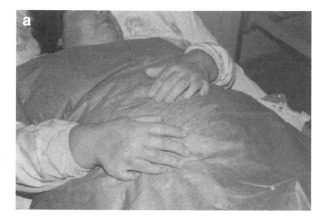
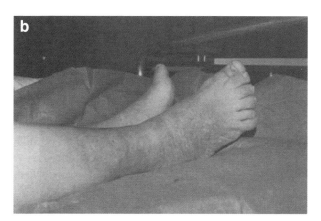

Figure 4.16 The Barbet–Biedl syndrome is a rare genetically transmitted form of syndromic obesity. These individuals have polydactyly, obesity and retinal abnormalities. There are several chromosomal locations associated with this syndrome and the gene for one of them has been identified. The other locations may be variants of the same enzyme. Reproduced with permission from Iannello S, Bosco P, Cavaleri A, et al. A review of the literature of Bardet–Biedl disease and report of three cases associated with metabolic syndrome and diagnosed after the age of fifty. *Obes Rev* 2002;3:123–35

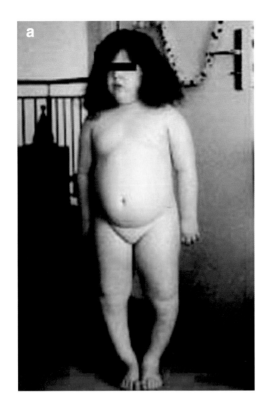

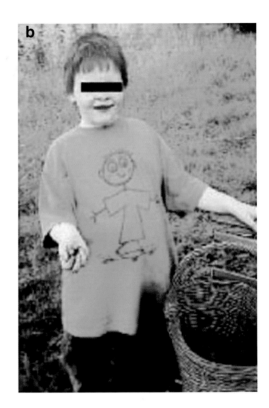

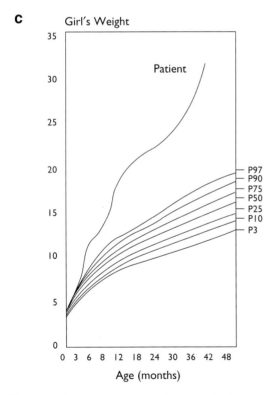

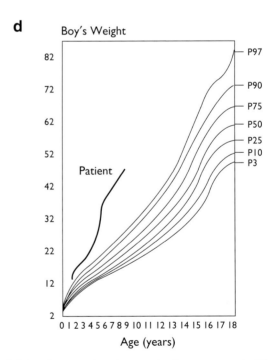

Figure 4.17 Picture and growth charts of a boy and girl who are deficient in pro-opiomelanocortin, the precursor to ACTH and α-MSH. This is a phenotypic form of obesity that can be recognized by the childhood onset of obesity and red hair, resulting from deficiency in α-melanocyte stimulating hormone. Reproduced with permission from Krude H, Biebermann H, Luck W, *et al*. Severe early-onset obesity, adrenal insufficiency and red hair pigmentation caused by POMC mutations in humans. *Nat Genet* 1998;19:155–7

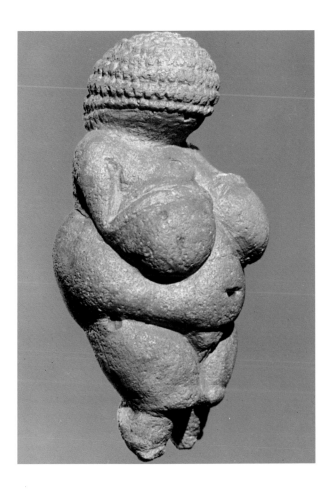

Figure 4.18 Venus of Willendorf is a stone age statue that indicates that obesity has been known to humans, possibly in the context of fertility, for more than 20 000 years (Vienna Museum of Natural History). This statue may be an example of the syndrome of progressive obesity, a name given to obesity that progresses year by year at the same absolute rate exceeding 4.5 kg/year. Since an increasing fat mass requires more energy, these individuals must have a progressive increase in energy intake and a persistent mismatch between intake and expenditure

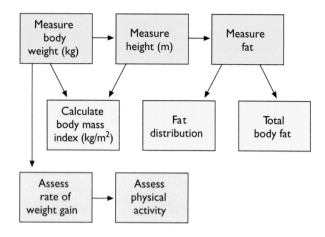

Figure 5.1 Patient encounter. The first step in a patient encounter with a health professional is to obtain information relevant to the problem with which the patient presents and other clinical problems. Obesity may play a role in the future health of the individual and its evaluation is the concern of this subsection

Figure 5.2 Natural history. Using the prevalence data for overweight for men and women, it is possible to identify three initial stages of the natural history of obesity. At birth, the entire population is pre-overweight, since at birth it is, for practical purposes, not possible to tell who will become overweight. As the years pass an increasing number of pre-overweight individuals become overweight and the pool of pre-overweight decreases. By the age of 60 when all of the potentially overweight individuals have become overweight it is possible to identify in retrospect a group of people who never became overweight

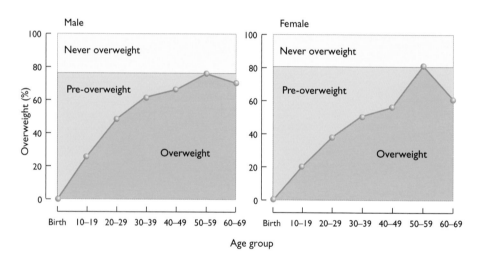

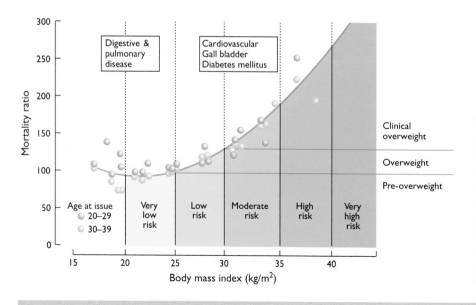

Figure 5.3 Using the relationship between mortality ratios from life insurance data on the predominantly Caucasian population we can identify pre-overweight, overweight and clinically overweight groups. Pre-overweight individuals will gradually become overweight and a segment of this group will progress to clinical overweight or clinical obesity

Risk factor	Defining level
Abdominal obesity (waist circumference)	
Men	< 102 cm (> 40 in)
Women	> 88 cm (> 35 in)
HDL-cholesterol	
Men	< 40 mg/dl
Women	> 50 mg/dl
Triglycerides	≥ 150 mg/dl
Fasting glucose	≥ 110 mg/dl
Blood pressure (SBP/DBP)	≥130/≥85 mmHg

Figure 5.4 The metabolic syndrome and insulin resistance are strongly related to central adiposity. However, insulin resistance is difficult to measure, so a variety of surrogate measures have been used to diagnose the metabolic syndrome. Criteria have been developed by the World Health Organization, the National Cholesterol Education Program in their Adult Treatment Panel III recommendations and by the American Association of Clinical Endocrinology. The clinical features of the metabolic syndrome listed below are those proposed by the Adult Treatment Panel III. The syndrome is present when an individual has three of these five criteria. In the United States population approximately 25% of adults have the metabolic syndrome. SBP, systolic blood pressure; DBP, diastolic blood pressure. Adapted with permission from National Cholesterol Education Program. Executive summary of the Third Report of The National Cholesterol Education Program (NCEP) Expert Panel on Detection, Evaluation and Treatment of High Blood Cholesterol in Adults (Adult Treatment Panel III). *J Am Med Assoc* 2001;285:2486–97, © 2001 American Medical Association

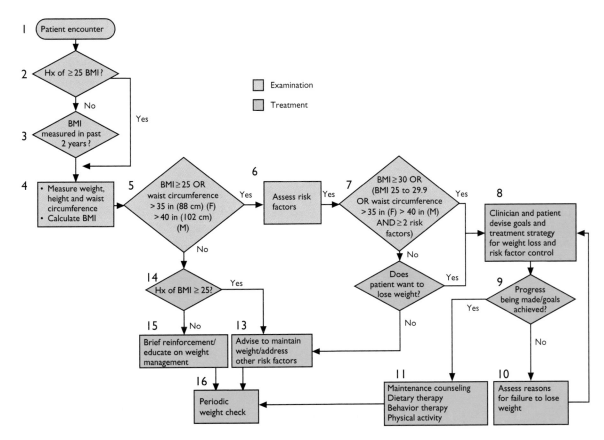

Figure 5.5 NHLBI algorithm for evaluating overweight. This figure shows the algorithm published by the NHLBI that can be used for evaluating overweight. It begins with the patient encounter and has the health professional measure height and weight to allow calculation of the body mass index (BMI) and waist circumference as an index of central fat. It then goes on to evaluate comorbidities and to develop a plan of action. Hx, history. Adapted with permission from NHLBI Obesity Education Initiative Expert Panel. Clinical guidelines on the identification, evaluation and treatment of overweight and obesity in adults – the evidence report. *Obes Res* 1998;6(Suppl. 2):51S–209S

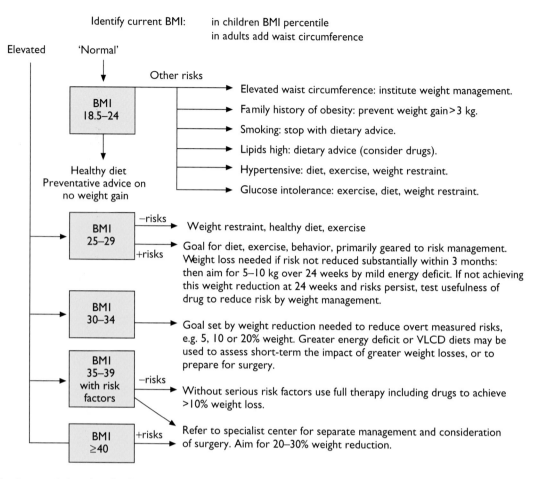

Figure 5.6   A second algorithm that I prefer is shown in this figure. It begins with the patient encounter which triggers the measurement of height and weight that are used to calculate the body mass index (BMI). This initial BMI needs adjustment based on ethnicity. For Asians, the upper acceptable limit is lowered to 23. For African-Americans and most Hispanics, it is raised to 26 or 27 kg/m². Thus the dividing line between normal and overweight can be shifted up or down depending on ethnic background. This encounter also triggers the evaluation of a variety of health risk factors. When BMI is within the normal range the patient/client can be given advice about a healthy diet and maintaining a healthy weight range. Medical concern shifts to the risk factors for cardiovascular disease and therapy is developed accordingly. All of these factors, except smoking, are considered in further evaluation of the BMI. These risk factors modify the selection of therapeutic choices as indicated in the overweight BMI group, and in the Obesity Class 2 group. VLCD, very low calorie diet. Adapted with permission from World Health Organization. *Obesity: Preventing and Managing the Glopal Epidemic. Report of a WHO Consultation.* Geneva: World Health Organization Technical Report Series No. 894, 2000

Predictors of weight gain
1. Parental overweight
2. Lower socioeconomic status
3. Smoking cessation
4. Low level of physical activity
5. High carbohydrate oxidation
6. Childhood overweight
7. Heavy babies
8. Lack of maternal knowledge of child's sweet eating habits
9. Recent marriage
10. Multiple births

Figure 5.7   Predictors of weight gain. A number of predictors have been identified that modify the risk for conversion from pre-overweight to overweight. After adjusting the initial body mass index (BMI) for ethnicity, individuals in the normal range should be evaluated for potential risks and advised accordingly

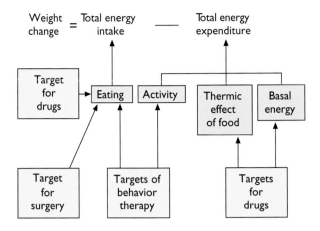

$$\text{Weight change} = \text{Total energy intake} \quad - \quad \text{Total energy expenditure}$$

Figure 5.8 An algorithm to approach selection of therapy. As noted in Section 2, obesity results from an imbalance between energy intake as food and energy expenditure as heat and work. This concept has been used here to show where the various therapeutic approaches are working

Risk-adjusted BMI	Category	Risk	Goal	Strategy
<25 → No	Pre-overweight →	Very low	Maintain weight	Healthy diet and exercise
25–29 → No	Preclinical overweight →	Low	Maintain or 5% weight loss	Exercise and healthy diet
30–34 → No	Clinical overweight →	Moderate	10% weight loss or BMI < 30	Medication Healthy diet Exercise
>35	Severe clinical overweight →	High	>15% weight loss or BMI reduction of >3 BMI units	Medication Healthy diet Exercise Surgery

Figure 5.9 Goals of therapy for adults. Preventing weight gain is the first goal for all body mass index (BMI) categories, except those with a BMI below 18.5 kg/m^2. Any weight loss can be viewed as a success and the magnitude of this success depends on the degree of loss

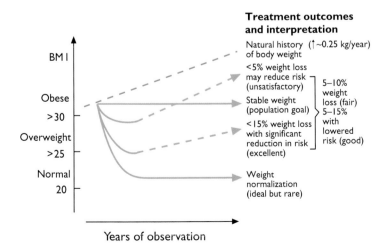

Figure 5.10 This figure shows various categories of success with weight loss programs. A loss of less than 5% after 1 year of treatment would be a failure. A loss between 5% and 10% that is maintained would be a limited success. A loss of < 10% would be an unqualified success although many people fantasize about reaching goals larger than this. Adapted with permission from Rossner S. Factors determining the long-term outcome of obesity treatment. In Bjorntorp P, Brodoff BN, eds. *Obesity*. Philadelphia: J.B. Lippincott Co, 1991: 712–9, © Lippincott Williams & Wilkins

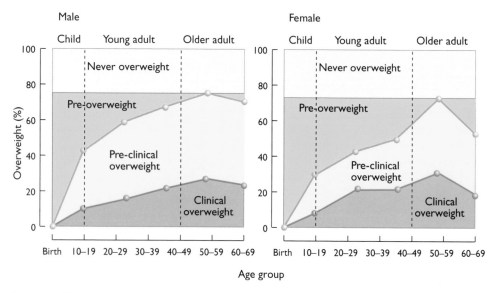

Figure 5.11 Using the natural history of obesity, we can divide the selection of treatments up according to stage of the problem and the age of the individual. This figure illustrates this approach

Age	Predictors of overweight	Therapeutic strategies		
		Pre-overweight at risk	Pre-clinical overweight	Clinical overweight
1–10	Positive family history Genetic defects (dysmorphic- PWS; Bardet-Biedl; Cohen) Hypothalamic injury Less than 3 months of nursing Diabetic or smoking mother	Family counseling Reduce inactivity	Family behavioral therapy Exercise Low fat– low energy- dense diet	Treat comorbidities Exercise Low fat– low energy- dense diet

Figure 5.12 Strategies for the treatment of children. The goal should be to prevent further excessive weight gain without impairing linear growth. Secondary goals should be to support the child's behavioral problems. Thus, family involvement is important. PWS, Prader–Willi syndrome

Age	Predictors of overweight	Therapeutic strategies		
		Pre-overweight at risk	Pre-clinical overweight	Clinical overweight
11–60	Positive family history of diabetes or obesity Endocrine disorders (PCO) Multiple pregnancies Marriage Smoking cessation Medication	Reduce sedentary lifestyle Low fat– low energy- dense diet Portion control	Behavior therapy Low fat– low energy- dense diet Reduce sedentary lifestyle	Treat comorbidities Drug treatment for overweight Reduce sedentary lifestyle Low fat– low energy- dense diet Behavior therapy Surgery

Figure 5.13 Strategies for adolescents and adults. As linear growth slows at puberty additional therapeutic strategies are possible and these individuals have many treatment strategies in common with adults. However, the adolescent culture is separate and deserves separate therapy

Age	Predictors of overweight	Therapeutic strategies		
		Pre-overweight at risk	Pre-clinical overweight	Clinical overweight
61–75	Menopause Declining growth hormone Declining testosterone Smoking cessation Medication	Few individuals remain in this subgroup	Behavior therapy Low fat–low energy-dense diet Reduce sedentary lifestyle	Treat comorbidities Drug treatment for overweight Reduce sedentary lifestyle Low fat–low energy-dense diet Behavior therapy Surgery

Figure 5.14 Strategies for older people when pre-overweight, and when preventive strategies are no longer a consideration

Imagined goal	Weight loss to achieve goal (kg(%))	% of subjects achieving goal
Dream weight	−37.4 (−38)	0%
Happy weight	−31.1 (−31)	9%
Acceptable weight	−24.9 (−25)	24%
Disappointed weight	−17.2 (−17)	20%
Below disappointed weight	—	47%

Baseline weight = 99.1 kg

Figure 5.15 Weight goals for overweight women. In this study women were asked to identify four categories of weight loss. The amount of weight loss that would put them at their 'Dream Weight'; an amount of weight loss that would make them 'Happy' but that was not their dream weight; an amount of weight loss that would be 'Acceptable' but that was less than their happy weight. Any weight loss less than this would be considered a disappointment. In this group of women, weight losses of less than 17.2% would leave them disappointed. Data derived from Foster GD, Wadden TA, Vogt RA, Brewer G. What is a reasonable weight loss? Patients' expectations and evaluations of obesity treatment outcomes. *J Consult Clin Psychol* 1997;65:79–85

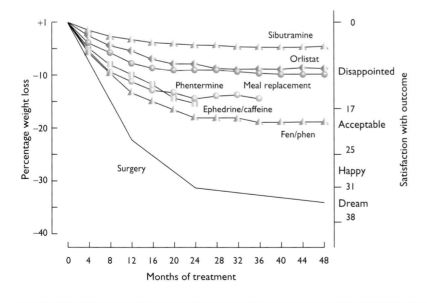

Figure 5.16 Relationship of weight loss by various treatments to imagined weight goals. This figure plots the weight loss curves for various therapeutic approaches including use of sibutramine, use of orlistat, use of meal replacement diets, use of combined drug therapy and surgical therapy. It is clear that only surgical therapy for obesity produced a weight loss that would produce a 'Dream Weight' for many individuals. The 'combination' therapy with drugs would be acceptable, but monotherapy would consistently produce only a disappointed level of weight loss. Thus in the patient encounter, the health professional and the patient need to come to an understanding of what level of weight loss is achievable

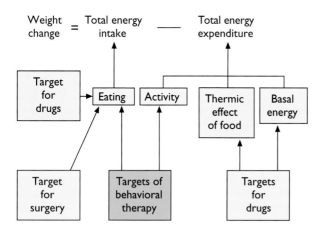

Figure 6.1   The targets of behavioral therapy in the energy balance diagram. Behavioral approaches to treating obesity tap into the fundamental mechanisms by which the brain consciously controls eating and physical activity

Component	Elements
Antecedents	The events that are associated with and that can serve as triggers for eating
Behaviors of eating	The time and place of eating The rate of eating The amount eaten
Consequences of eating	Using rewards for modifying antecedents and eating behaviors such as point systems

Figure 6.2   The ABC Scheme for evaluating behavioral strategies to control obesity. The 'A' stands for the antecedents of eating, the 'B' for the behavior of eating itself and the 'C' for the consequences of eating

Most helpful behavioral techniques

1. Self-monitoring
2. Stimulus control
3. Stress management
4. Cognitive behavioral strategies
5. Contingency management

Figure 6.3   This table indicates which of the behavioral approaches are the most useful in helping to keep weight off

Behavioral predictors of weight loss

1. Positive feelings
2. Internal motivation
3. Focusing on positive changes in health, fitness and appearance
4. Social support

Figure 6.4   Behavior therapy is now a main component of most weight loss programs. Its use is recommended in the NHLBI report on obesity and they give it an evidence level of B which means the evidence for its value is strong, but not the strongest

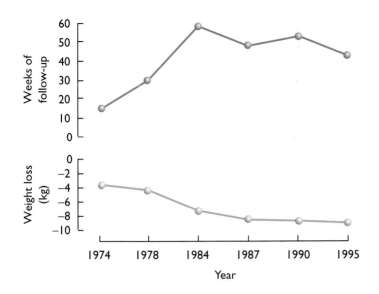

Figure 6.5 The improving success of behavioral therapy over time. The characteristics of behavioral programs for the treatment of obesity have changed over time. The programs have become longer in duration, and as a result they have increased the degree of weight loss. This shown from the summary of a number of recent studies. Data derived from Williamson DA, Perrin LA. Behavioral therapy for obesity. *Endocrinol Metab Clin North Am* 1996;25:943–54

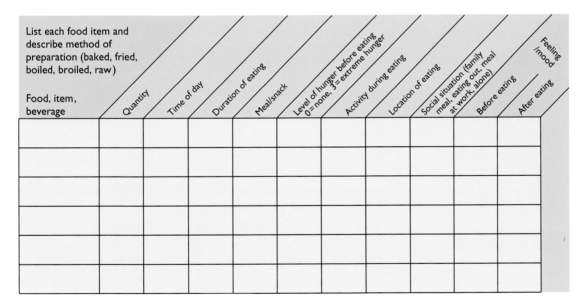

Figure 6.6 To monitor the conditions that affect obesity and the behavior itself requires a process. The original process recorded all of the facets of the eating behavior on a single form

a   Physician's diet plan: Monitor of associated activity

Day: _____	
Food eaten	Associated activity

Physician's diet plan: Analysis of associated activity

	1	2	3	4	5	6	7	8	9	10	11	12	13	14	Add'l	Total
Reading	■	■	■	■	■											5
Watching TV	■	■	■													3
Preparing meal	■	■														2
Talking	■	■	■													3
None	■	■	■	■												4
Other																
Other	■	■														2

b   Physician's diet plan: Monitor for places of eating

Day: _____	
Food eaten	Place

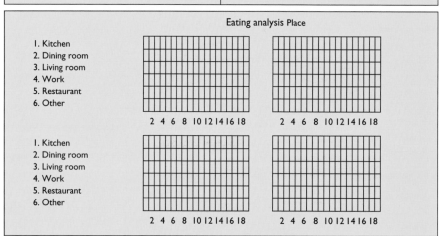

Eating analysis Place

1. Kitchen
2. Dining room
3. Living room
4. Work
5. Restaurant
6. Other

2 4 6 8 10 12 14 16 18   2 4 6 8 10 12 14 16 18

1. Kitchen
2. Dining room
3. Living room
4. Work
5. Restaurant
6. Other

2 4 6 8 10 12 14 16 18   2 4 6 8 10 12 14 16 18

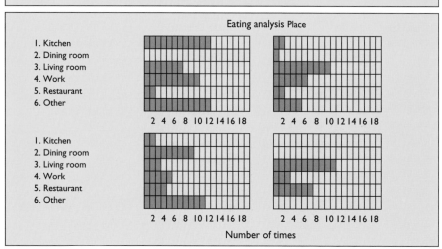

Eating analysis Place

1. Kitchen
2. Dining room
3. Living room
4. Work
5. Restaurant
6. Other

2 4 6 8 10 12 14 16 18   2 4 6 8 10 12 14 16 18

1. Kitchen
2. Dining room
3. Living room
4. Work
5. Restaurant
6. Other

2 4 6 8 10 12 14 16 18   2 4 6 8 10 12 14 16 18

Number of times

Figure 6.7 A second approach to monitoring behavior uses forms for individual behaviors (a and b). The forms for recording the places of eating and the frequency of eating events is shown. During the week between meetings, individuals record on 3 × 5 cards one of these events. At the next session they analyze what they have recorded by marking on recording forms to obtain results like those shown here. The next week they take another behavior and record again what they have done and then analyze it at the next meeting

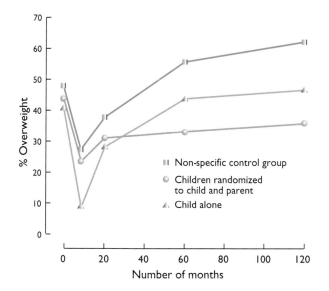

Figure 6.8 Long-term effectiveness of behavioral skills in reducing future weight of children has been demonstrated in a ten-year study. Overweight children aged 6–12 were included in behavioral weight programs in three settings. The first included the child and the parent together. The second included the child and the parent, but in separate treatment groups, and the third was a control group. Ten years after the treatment, the child treated with the parent maintained significantly more of the weight loss than those in the other two groups. Adapted with permission from Epstein LH, Valoski A, Wing RR, McCurley J. Ten-year follow-up of behavioral, family-based treatment for obese children. *J Am Med Assoc* 1990;264:2519–23, ©1990 American Medical Association

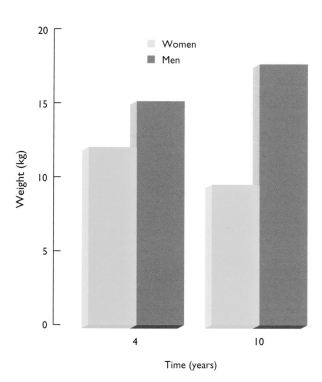

Figure 6.9 A ten-year study of behavioral therapy in Sweden has shown that with continued treatment weight can be kept lower than baseline. The initial treatment compared a short hospitalization and behavioral therapy with a group that had jaw-wiring (dental fixation). The dentally fixed group lost more weight, but when the wires were removed weight regain was rapid. In the group treated with behavioral strategies many patients maintained a long-term weight loss. Data derived from Bjorvell H, Rossner S. A ten-year follow-up of weight change in severely obese subjects treated in a combined behavioural modification programme. *Int J Obes Relat Metab Disord* 1992;16: 623–5

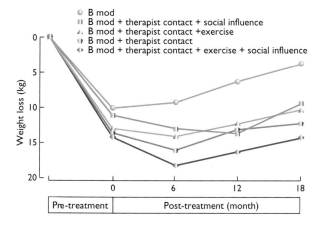

Figure 6.10 The intensity of the behavioral strategies also improves weight loss. As the number of modalities that are used is increased, subjects lose and maintain more of the weight loss. Data derived from Perri MG, Sears SF Jr, Clark JE. Strategies for improving maintenance of weight loss. Toward a continuous care model of obesity management. *Diabetes Care* 1993;16:200–9

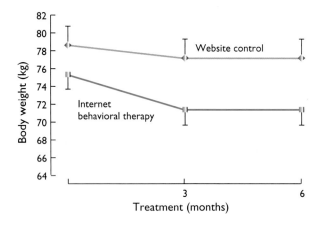

Figure 6.11 The internet is the latest tool applied to behavioral therapy. This figure shows that a behavioral program administered over the internet produces significantly more weight loss than access to an informational website without behavioral techniques being implemented. Adapted with permission from Tate DF, Wing RR, Winett RA. Using internet technology to deliver a behavioral weight loss program. *J Am Med Assoc* 2001;285:1172–7, © 2001 American Medical Association

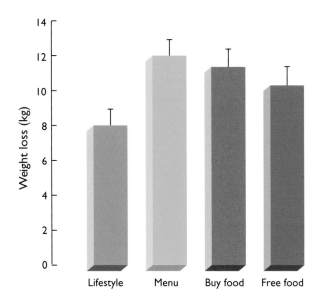

Figure 6.12 Adding a structural eating plan to a behavioral plan can also improve weight loss. In this study either menus, providing free food and a structured eating plan enhanced the magnitude of weight loss. Wing RR, Jeffery RW, Burton LR, *et al.* Food provision versus structured meal plans in the behavioral treatment of obesity. *Int J Obes Relat Metab Disord* 1996; 20:56–62

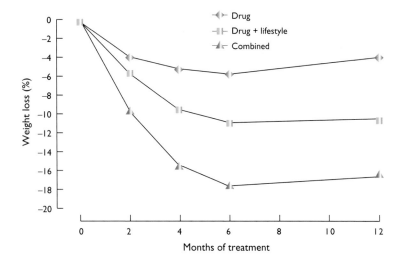

Figure 6.13 Adding behavioral strategies to drug treatment also improves weight loss. In this trial all patients were treated with sibutramine. Adding behavioral therapy or behavioral therapy and a structured meal plan produced significantly more weight loss. Adapted with permission from Wadden TA, Berkowitz RI, Sarwer DB, *et al.* Benefits of lifestyle modification in the pharmacologic treatment of obesity: a randomized trial. *Arch Intern Med* 2001;161:218–27

Physician's diet plan: Analysis of pre-planning, number of times

	Number of times															
	1	2	3	4	5	6	7	8	9	10	11	12	13	14	Add'l	Total
Food item eaten, not planned																
Food item planned, not eaten																
More food eaten than planned																
Less food eaten than planned																
Eating at time/place not planned																
Ate as planned (gold star)																

Physician's diet plan: Analysis of pre-planning, number of times

	Number of times															
	1	2	3	4	5	6	7	8	9	10	11	12	13	14	Add'l	Total
Food item eaten, not planned	▓															
Food item planned, not eaten	▓	▓														
More food eaten than planned	▓															
Less food eaten than planned	▓															
Eating at time/place not planned	▓	▓	▓													
Ate as planned (gold star)	▓	▓	▓	▓												

Figure 6.14 Learning to control eating events takes planning. This figure shows a form that can be printed on a 3 × 5 card that allows identifying times when planned food is eaten

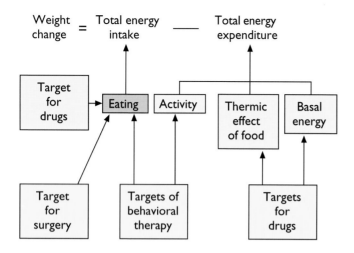

Figure 7.1 Identification of the site at which diet works to influence energy balance. It reduces total energy intake and can in turn be influenced by other strategies

a

Type of diet
Low fat diets (< 20% fat)
Low carbohydrate diets (< 100 g/day)
Balanced low calorie diets
Diets focused on one type of food

b

Characterization of diets in absolute amount (grams)				
Type of diet	Total kcals	Fat g (%)	Carbohydrate g (%)	Protein g (%)
Typical American	2200	85 (35)	275 (50)	82.5 (15)
High-fat, low-carbohydrate	1414*	94 (60)	35 (10)	105 (30)
Moderate-fat, balanced nutrient reduction	1450	40 (25)	218 (60)	54 (15)
Low- and very-low fat	1450	16 – 24 (10 – 15)	235 –271 (65 – 75)	54 – 72 (15 – 20)

*Based on average intake of subjects who self-selected low carbohydrate diets.

Figure 7.2 A classification of diets based on energy levels (a and b). Diets are either low or very low in energy. This is accomplished by modifying the foods differently. For the very low calorie diets, formulas are often used. The other diets are a balanced reduction in calories, a reduction in carbohydrates, a reduction in fat or a focus on specific foods. (b) Adapted with permission from Friedman MR, King J, Kennedy E. Popular diets: a scientific review. *Obes Res* 2001;9(Suppl. 1):1S–40S

Revised WHO equations for estimating basal metabolic rate (BMR)		
Men		
18 – 30 years = (0.0630 x actual weight in kg + 2.8957) x 240 kcal/day		
31 – 60 years = (0.0484 x actual weight in kg + 3.6534) x 240 kcal/day		
Women		
18 – 30 years = (0.0621 x actual weight in kg + 2.0357) x 240 kcal/day		
31 – 60 years = (0.0342 x actual weight in kg + 3.5377) x 240 kcal/day		
Estimated total		
Energy expenditure = BMR x activity factor		
Activity level	**Activity factor**	
Low (sedentary)	1.3	
Intermediate (some regular exercise)	1.5	
High (regular activity or demanding job)	1.7	

Figure 7.3 To reduce calories as a strategy to lose weight, we must have an estimate for energy needs. The formula for estimating energy recommended by the World Health Organization/Food and Agricultural Organization of the United Nations is widely used and is shown above

Physician's diet plan: Monitor for calories

Day: _____				
Food eaten	Amount (weight)		Calories	
			Solid	Liquid

Physician's diet plan: Analysis of caloric intake

	1	2	3	4	5	6	7	Grand total
Solid								
Liquid								
Sum								

Physician's diet plan: Analysis of caloric intake

	1	2	3	4	5	6	7	Grand total
Solid	1200	1000	1500	1450	1550	1000	1250	8950
Liquid	200	150	300	100	150	100	150	1150
Sum	1400	1150	1800	1550	1700	1100	1400	10 100

Figure 7.4 As part of the strategy for behavioral control, a form for recording calories and for analysing the data was developed. The calories for foods were obtained from standard calorie books. Portion size was estimated and the calories eaten at each meal for each item were recorded. They were then averaged for each day in the liquid and solid form to obtain the entire week's value. Liquid calories (alcohol and sugar-containing beverages) were separated because they can be a problem in their own right and separable from the calories in solid food

Nutrition facts		
Serving size 8 fl oz (240 ml)		
Servings per container 8		
Amount per serving		
Calories 100	Calories from fat 20	
	% Daily value*	
Total fat 2.5g		4%
Saturated fat 1.5g		8%
Cholesterol 10mg		3%
Sodium 130mg		5%
Total carbohydrate 12g		4%
Dietary fiber 0g		0%
Sugars 11g		
Protein 8g		
Vitamin A 10g	•	Vitamin C 4%
Calcium 30g	•	Iron 0%
Vitamin D 25g		

*Percent daily values are based on a 2000 calorie diet. Your daily values may be higher or lower depending on your calorie needs:

	Calories	2000	2500
Total fat	less than	65g	80g
Saturated fat	less than	20g	25g
Cholesterol	less than	300mg	300mg
Sodium	less than	2400mg	2400mg
Total carbohydrate		300g	375g
Dietary fiber		25g	30g

Ingredients: Low-fat milk, vitamin A palmitate, vitamin D₃

Figure 7.5 The nutrition label for low-fat milk. The food label is a good source of information about calories and nutrition. A typical label is shown here illustrating information for low-fat milk. At the top are the calories per serving and then the number of servings per package and the percent of these calories that come from fat. This information can be used as one tool for tracking calorie intake

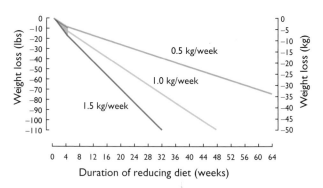

Figure 7.6 A deficit of 500 kcal/day will produce about 0.5 kg weight loss per week, depending on the individual's weight. This figure shows the duration of dieting required for 0.5 kg/week, 1.0 kg/week or 1.5 kg/week weight loss which is about 500, 1000 or 1500 kcal/day deficit

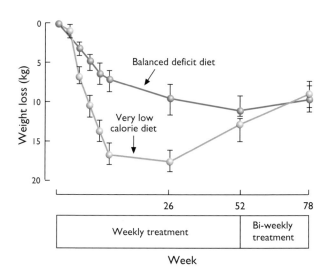

Figure 7.7 Comparison of a balanced deficit diet and a very low calorie diet shows that the initial loss with the very low calorie diet is greater, but that over time the weight loss of the two groups gradually converges. Adapted with permission from Wadden TA, Foster GE, Letizia KA. One-year behavioral treatment of obesity: comparison of moderate and severe caloric restriction and the effects of weight maintenance therapy. *J Consult Clin Psychol* 1994;62:165–71, ©1994 American Psychological Association

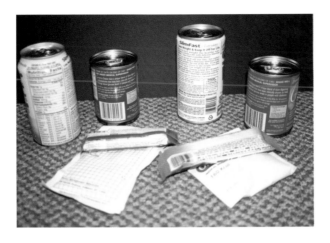

Figure 7.8 Portion control is a good strategy to control energy intake. This can be done with formula diets, with frozen foods or with food bars. Examples of some of the formula diets and frozen foods that have been developed are depicted in this photograph

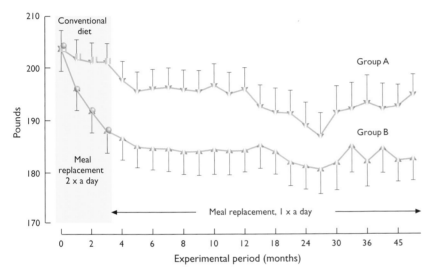

Figure 7.9 Weight loss with meal replacements has been studied over 4 years. In group A subjects received a conventional diet for the first three months followed by one meal replacement for the remainder of the time. The subjects in group B had two meal replacements for for the first 3 months followed by a single one for 48 months. It is clear that portion-control using meal replacements can be beneficial in inducing weight loss and in helping maintain it. Structured meal plans, including portion control have been used to enhance weight loss with a behavioral weight control program (see Figure 6.8). Adapted with permission from Flechtner-Mors M, Ditschuneit HH, Johnson TD, et al. Metabolic and weight loss effects of long-term dietary intervention in obese patients: four-year results. *Obes Res* 2000;8:399–402

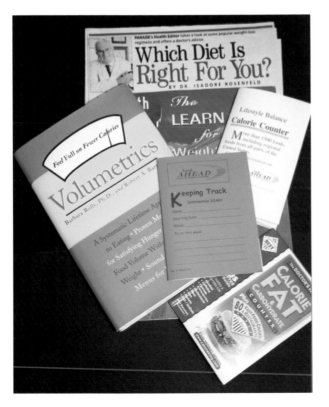

Figure 7.10 Calorie counters, fat gram counters and diet books. High-fat levels in the diet increase the risk of developing obesity in some people. Fat counting is an alternative to counting calories and to portion control where the manufacturer counts the calories. Guides with fat grams are readily available and they can form an alternative or complementary strategy for weight loss. Many diet books are also available

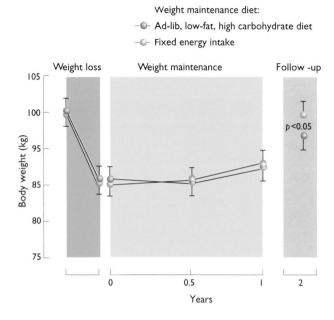

Weight maintenance diet:
- Ad-lib, low-fat, high carbohydrate diet
- Fixed energy intake

Figure 7.11 A low-fat diet ad-lib had a slightly better effect on the prevention of weight regain after an initial weight loss than a low-calorie diet. Adapted with permission from Toubro S, Astrup A. Randomized comparison of diets for maintaining obese subjects' weight after major weight loss: ad lib, low fat, high carbohydrate diet versus fixed energy intake. *Br Med J* 1997;314:29–34

Duration of breast feeding at school entry	Prevalence of obesity at school entry
at school entry	4.5%
3 months	3.8%
3–5 months	2.3%
6–12 months	1.7%
>12 months	0.8%

Figure 7.12 Prolonged breast feeding can reduce the prevalence of overweight at entry into school. In this study there was a graded reduction in percent of overweight children entering school as the length of breast feeding increased. Data derived from Von Kries R, Koletzko B, Sauerwald T, *et al*. Breast feeding and obesity: cross-sectional study. *Br Med J* 1999;319:147–50

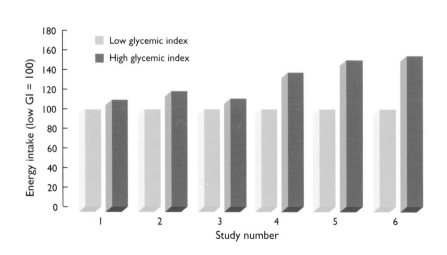

Figure 7.13 The rate at which glucose is released from starch can be used to calculate a 'glycemic index' (GI). Potato and rice are readily digested and absorbed and can be used to relate other starches. As the fiber in a diet increases the rate of release of glucose is slowed producing food with a 'low' glycemic index. In a review of these foods Roberts produced data showing that energy intake as food was increased with food of a high glycemic index. Data derived from Roberts SB. High-glycemic index foods, hunger and obesity: is there a connection? *Nutr Rev* 2000;58:163–9

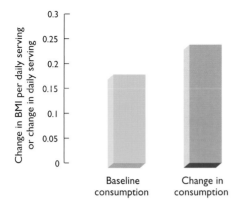

Figure 7.14 The consumption of sugar-sweetened beverages in children was associated with an increasing BMI in children suggesting increased fattening. This may be due to the sweet taste of the high fructose corn sweeteners (see Figure 2.11). Data derived from Ludwig DS, Peterson KE, Gortmaker SL. Relation between consumption of sugar-sweetened drinks and childhood obesity: a prospective, observational analysis. *Lancet* 2001;357:505–8

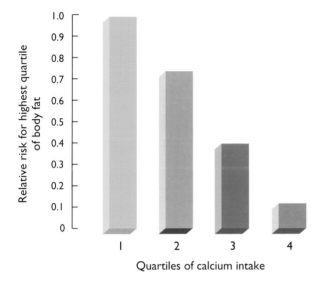

Figure 7.15 Calcium intake and body weight. Cross-sectional studies show that higher calcium intake is associated with lower body weight (Zemel MB, Shi H, Great B, *et al.* Regulation of adiposity by dietary calcium. *FASEB J* 2000;14:1132–8). Feeding studies also show that body weight decreases as the amount of supplemental calcium in the diet is increased (Davies KM, Heaney RP, Recker RR, *et al.* Calcium intake and body weight. *J Clin Endocrinol Metab* 2000;85:4635–8)

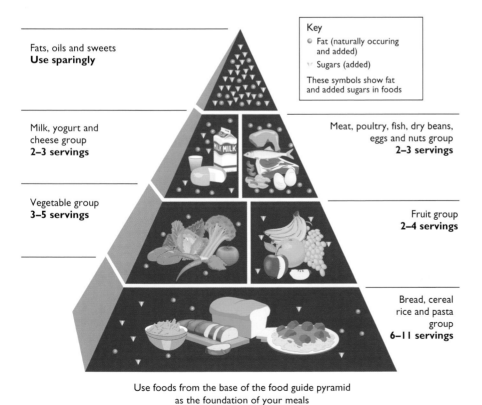

Figure 7.16 The food guide pyramid. The food guide pyramid provides a structure for selecting foods. At the bottom are the whole grains, breads and cereals. Above them are the fruits and vegetables and above that the meats, cheeses and dairy products with the recommended range of servings for each

Food Group	Relative calorie (energy) value				
	Low		High		
Bread and Cereal **(6–11 servings)**	Bread Melba toast Dry non-sugared cereals Cooked grain cereals		Biscuits Muffins Rolls Cornbread and grits Crackers Cookies Pie Pasta (macaroni, noodles, etc.) Tortillas Doughnuts		

Vegetables and fruit
 	
(2–5 servings)
	Asparagus
	Beets
	Broccoli
	Cabbage
	Celery
	Chard-spinach
	Cucumber
	Green beans
	Greens
	Lettuce
	Mushrooms
	Pickles
	  (dill or sour)
	Summer squash
	Tomatoes
	Turnips
	Winter squash
		Apple juice
		Apricots
		Cantaloupe
		Berries
		Boysenberries
		Cranberries
		Lemon
		Gooseberries
		Grapefruit
		Oranges
		Papayas
		Peaches
		Strawberries
		Watermelon
			Lima beans
			Peas
			Potatoes
			Sweet
			  potatoes
				Apples
				Bananas
				Cherries
				Grape juice
				Guava
				Mango
				Pears
				Pineapple
				Plums
				Prunes
				Raspberries
					50 kcal/
					100 g raw
					vegetable
					or fruit

Milk, yogurt and cheese (2 servings for adults (3 servings for children)	Skim milk Low-fat milk Buttermilk Yogurt (skim milk – without fruit)		Cottage cheese Whole milk Ice cream Evaporated milk Goat milk Cheese		60 kcal/ 100g

Meat, fish, poultry and dry beans
 	
(2–3 servings)
	Liver
	Chicken
	Shell fish,
	  (shrimp,
	  crab, clams,
	  oyster,
	  lobster)
		Abalone
		Bass
		Cod
		Flounder
		Pike
		Halibut (Calif)
		Swordfish
		Tuna
		  (water pack)
		Haddock
		Perch
		Trout (brook)
			Beef
			Ham
			Lamb
			Pork
			Bologna
			Hot dogs
			Turkey
			Veal
			Egg
				Herring
				  (Atlantic)
				Sardines
				Trout
				  (Rainbow)
				Tuna
				  (oil pack)
				Salmon
				Whitefish
					150kcal/
					100g raw

Figure 7.17 This table lists food groups in relation to calories, with foods with more energy for a given weight shown on the right and those with less energy for a given weight on the left. As a food selection strategy, you are better advised to select foods from the left-hand portion of the table

		Men	Women
Energy (19–50 yr)	Kca/kg (kJ)	2900	2200
Protein (19–50 yr)	g	0.8	0.8
Calcium	mg	800	800
Magnesium	mg	350	280
Phosphorus	mg	800	800
Iron	mg	10	15
Zinc	mg	15	12
Iodine	mcg	—	150
Selenium	mcg	70	55
Vitamin A	(mcgRE)	900	700
Vitamin D	mcg	10	10
Vitamin E	(mg α-TE)	10	8
Vitamin K	mcg	80	65
Thiamin	mg	1.5	1.1
Riboflavin	mg	1.7	1.3
Niacin	mg	19	15
Vitamin B_6	mg	2.0	1.6
Vitamin B_{12}	mg	2.0	2.0
Vitamin C	mcg	60	60
Folate	mcg	200	180

Figure 7.18 Recommended dietary intake of selected nutrients for men and women

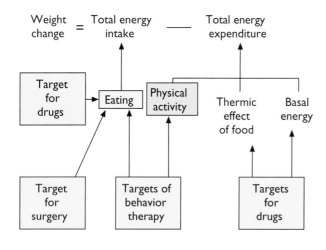

Figure 8.1 The relation of physical activity to the energy balance equation is shown here. It is important to remember that physical activity expends energy, but that a significant part of physical activity is the 'cognitive' decision to be active. Thus, physical activity and plans to increase activity are an important part of strategies for behavior modification

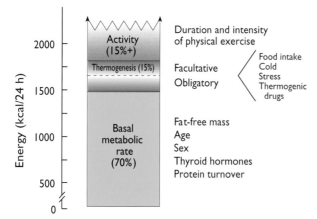

Figure 8.2 The relation of physical activity and energy expenditure to the total daily energy expenditure is illustrated in this figure. Although physical activity is 'open-ended' in reality it almost always ranges between 1.4 and 1.7 times the resting metabolic rate

	in food	Calories (54.5 kg)	120 lb (73 kg)	160 lb (91 kg)
		Minutes to burn calories, walking at 3 mph		
Apple (1) (2.1" diam)	75	21	17	14
Apple pie (1/6 of 9" pie)	410	115	93	78
Beer (12 oz)	170	47	38	31
Blueberries (cup, fresh)	87	23	19	16
Beef steak (cubed, 4 oz)	300	83	68	57
Bologna (1 sl)	88	23	19	22
Biscuit (1, 2" diam)	130	36	30	24
Bread (1 sl)	65	18	15	12
Broccoli (cup)	50	14	12	10
Cola (8 oz, Coke)	100	28	23	19
Cereal (cooked, cup)	165	46	38	31
Cheese (1 oz, gouda, caraway)	100	28	23	19
Chocolate cake (1 piece) (2 x 3 x 2", no icing)	165	46	38	31
Egg (medium)	78	22	18	15
Flounder (4 oz, raw)	78	22	18	15
Frankfurter	124	34	28	23
Hamburger & bun (1 bun, 3 oz high-fat meat)	400	111	91	76
Milk (whole, 8 oz)	166	46	38	31
Orange (large, 3-3/8" diam)	115	32	27	23
Potato (1, baked, no skin, 2-1/2" diam)	100	28	23	19
Salmon (canned, 31 oz)	200	56	46	38
Strawberries (cup)	54	15	12	10

Figure 8.3 Energy in food is expended in basal energy needs and in activity. This table shows the calorie values in a few food items and the amount of time required to burn these calories for people of different weights. Since heavier people expend more energy to move their body, they need to spend less time to utilize the energy in any given food as is shown in this figure

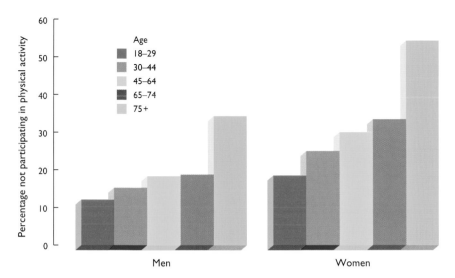

Figure 8.4 People in affluent countries are relatively inactive physically. This is shown in the Surgeon General's report from the United States. Here the percentage not participating in physical activity increases with age, a finding that correlates with the increasing prevalence of overweight and obesity. Data derived from US Department of Health and Human Services. *Physical Activity and Health: A Report of the Surgeon General.* Atlanta, GA: National Center for Chronic Disease Prevention and Health Promotion, 1996

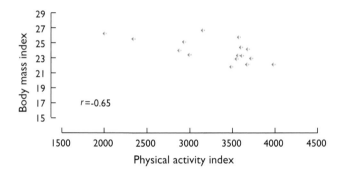

Figure 8.5 The relation of inactivity to body mass index (BMI) is shown in an epidemological study. As the physical activity index increases the average BMI declined. Adapted with permission from Kromhout D, Bloemberg B. Seidell JC, *et al.* Physical activity and dietary fiber determine polulation body fat levels: the Seven Countries Study. *Int J Obes Relat Metab Disord* 2001;25:301–6

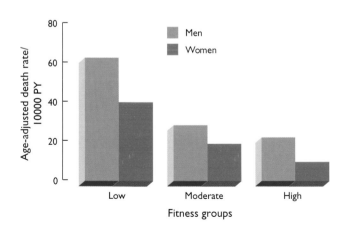

Figure 8.6 A regular pattern of physical activity can reduce the risk of premature death. In this figure both men and women had lower death rates as their level of physical activity increased from low to high. Data derived from Blair SN, Kohl HW III, Paffenbarger RS, *et al.* Physical fitness and all-cause mortality. A prospective study of healthy men and women. *J Am Med Assoc* 1989;262:2395–401

a

Heart rates (beats/minute) accordng to age*				
Age (years)	55% of maximum[a]	60% of maximum[b]	90% of maximum[c]	maximum[d]
20	110	120	180	200
25	107	117	177	195
30	104	114	173	190
35	102	111	168	185
40	99	108	163	180
45	96	105	159	175
50	93	102	153	170
55	91	99	149	165
60	88	96	143	160
65	85	93	140	155
70	82	90	135	150
75	80	87	132	145
80	77	84	129	140

*This formula is only an approximation of any individual's response and will not apply when certain rate-altering medications are being taken, such as β-blockers and some calcium antagonists.

a Minimum exercise heart rate for health benefit designated by ACSM.

b Minimum exercise heart rate for fitness designated by ACSM.

c Maximum exercise heart rate designated by ACSM.

d Maximum average heart rate adjusted for age (according to formula: maximum = 220 − age).

b

	Apparently healthy		Higher risk[a]		
Medical examination and diagnostic exercise test recommended prior to:	Age ≤ 40 years (men) ≤ 50 years (women)	Age > 40 years (men) > 50 years (women)	No Symptoms	Symptoms	With disease[b]
Moderate exercise[c]	no	no	no	yes	yes
Vigorous exercise[d]	no	yes	yes	yes	yes

a Individuals with 2 or more coronary risk factors or symptoms

b Individuals with known cardiac, pulmonary, or metabolic disease

c Moderate exercise – exercise intensity well within the individual's current capacity and that can be comfortably sustained for a prolonged period of time (i.e. 60 mins); slow progression and generally uncompetitive

d Vigorous exercise – exercise intense enough to represent a substantial challenge and that would ordinarily result in fatigue within 20 min

Figure 8.7 When doing aerobic activity, the heart rate rises as shown here in (a). The maximal rise is related to age. As a guide, heart rate should increase to more than 50% of the maximum, but not above 80%. Warming up for 5 min and then cooling down with slow activity is advisable at the beginning and end of an exercise program. (b) Guidelines for medical examinations and diagnostic exercise tests prior to exercise. Adapted with permission from American College of Sports Medicine, Preventive and Rehabilitative Exercise Committee. *Guidelines: for Exercise Testing and Prescription*, 4th edn. Philadelphia, PA: Lea & Febiger, 1991, © Lea & Febiger

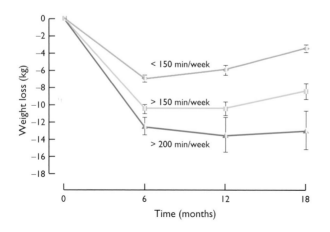

Figure 8.8 Exercise can increase weight loss, and the weight loss is related to the amount of the exercise. However, for overweight individuals there is the risk of injury to joints and tendons with vigorous exercise. I only recommend an increase in walking that is an activity that everyone is able to undertake. When more vigorous activity is contemplated it is desirable for many people to have a cardiac stress test beforehand to make sure there is no cardiac disease. Adapted with permission from Jakicic JM, Winters C, Lang W, Wing RR. Effects of intermittent exercise and use of home exercise equipment on adherence, weight loss and fitness in overweight women: a randomized trial. *J Am Med Assoc* 1999;282:1554–60, © 1999 American Medical Association

Variable	Diet (D)[a]	Exercise (E)[a]	Diet + Exercise (DE)[a]
Weight loss (kg)	10.7 ± 0.5 (269)	2.9 ± 0.4*, **, ***, **** (90)	11.0 ± 0.6 (134)
Percentage body fat decrease	6.0 ± 1.0 (46)	3.5 ± 0.5*, ***, **** (56)	7.3 ± 0.8 (43)
Weight loss maintained at 1 year[b]	6.6 ± 0.5 (91)	6.1 ± 2.1 (7)	8.6 ± 0.8 (54)

Data are means ± S.E.M.
*Significantly different from other program types when ANOVA was run without covariates
**Significantly different from other program types when analysis was run with initial body weight as a covariate
***Significantly different from other program types when analysis was run with initial percentage body fat as a covariate
****Significantly different from other program types when analysis was run with initial body mass index (BMI) as a covariate

a Number in parenthesis represents the number of studies reporting data for this particular variable (this number may be varied for the covariate analyses if a study did not report data for the covariate in question)
b Not enough studies included data for a covariate analysis using initial percentage body fat or initial BMI as the covariate

Figure 8.9 Exercise as a single modality for the treatment of obesity is not very effective. A meta-analysis of diet and exercise programs showed that weight loss with exercise alone averaged about 1.5 kg versus 5.5 kg for diet alone and a small additional effect of combining the two

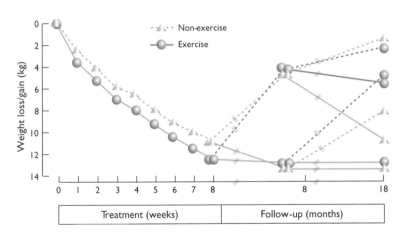

Figure 8.10 Exercise is a useful strategy for preventing weight regain. At the end of this treatment program there was little difference between the groups with and without exercise. However, in the men who maintained an ongoing exercise program, or who re-instituted an exercise program later after a weight gain there was better maintenance of the lower weight than when exercise was discontinued. Adapted with permission from Pavlou KN, Krey S, Steffee SP. Exercise as an adjunct to weight loss and maintenance in moderately obese subjects. *Am J Clin Nutr* 1989;49:1115–23, © American Journal of Clinical Nutrition/ American Society for Clinical Nutrition

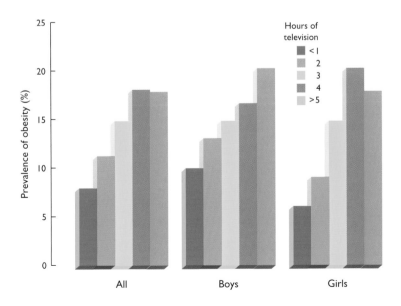

Figure 8.11 Time spent viewing television is related to the degree of overweight in children. In this study by the National Center for Health Statistics on 8–16-year-olds there was a graded increase in weight and food intake with increasing time spent watching television. Adapted with permission from Crespo CH, Smit E, Troiano RP, *et al.* Television watching, energy intake, and obesity in US children: results from the third National Health and Nutrition Examination Survey, 1988–1994. *Arch Pediatr Adolesc Med* 2001;155:360–5

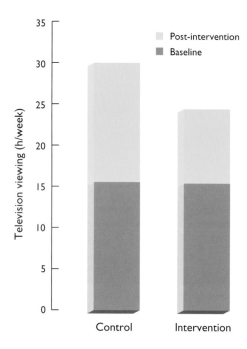

Figure 8.12 In a school-based program children in the intervention group that reduced television watching time gained less weight than the children in the control group that did not reduce television watching. Data derived from Robinson TN. Reducing children's television viewing to prevent obesity: a randomized controlled trial. *J Am Med Assoc* 1999; 282:1561–7

Activity	NHIS Percent reporting activity		NWCR	
	M	**F**	**M**	**F**
Walking	39.4%	48.3%	78.6%	76.1%
Running	12.8%	5.7%	20.4%	8.2%
Cycling	16.2%	14.6%	22.4%	20.2%
Aerobics	2.8%	11.1%	4.1%	20.9%
Stair climbing	9.9%	11.6%	3.1%	9.5%
Weight lifting	20.0%	8.8%	24.0%	19.5%

Figure 8.13 People who are successful in losing weight maintain a higher level of activity. This is shown in people who have maintained weight loss in the National Weight Control Registry. NHIS, National Health Interview Survey 1991; NWCR, National Weight Control Registry. Data derived from McGuire MT, Wing RR, Klem ML, Hill JO. Behavioral strategies of individuals who have maintained long-term weight losses. *Obes Res* 1999;7:334–41

Activity	Calories burned per hour
Shopping	150
Dancing	250
House cleaning, scrubbing, vacuuming	227
Walking (4 mph)	312

Two-thirds of body weight expressed in calories/mile walking or running is a way to express energy expenditure in relation to body size.

Figure 8.14 This table shows the energy expenditure associated with some common daily activities. Normally we spend about 1 kcal/min at rest. As we increase the degree of activity this can rise to several calories per minute. This figure includes both the basal- and activity-related energy

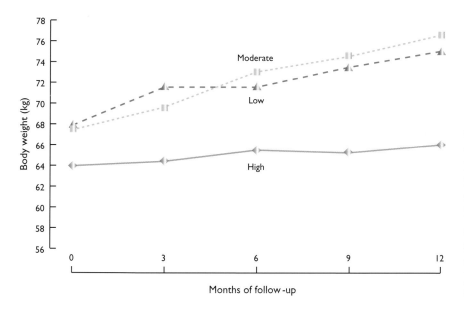

Figure 8.15 This figure shows the amount of energy that must be expended to maintain a weight loss in individuals who have previously lost weight. Adapted with permission from Schoeller DA, Shay K, Kushner RF. How much physical activity is needed to minimize weight gain in previously obese women? *Am J Clin Nutr* 1997;66:551–6, © American Journal of Clinical Nutrition/American Society for Clinical Nutrition

Body weight		Energy expended (kcal)	
pounds	kg	5000 steps	10000 steps
88	40	100	200
110	50	125	250
132	60	150	300
154	70	175	350
176	80	200	400
198	90	225	450
220	100	250	500

Figure 8.16 Walking is an ideal method of exercise for overweight individuals. This table shows the amount of energy expended for different numbers of steps and the amount of energy expended as the body weight increases

Date	Drug	Outcome
1893	Thyroid	Hyperthyroidism
1933	Dinitrophenol	Cataracts, neuropathy
1937	Amphetamine	Addiction
1967	Rainbow pills (digitalis, diuretics)	Deaths
1971	Aminorex	Pulmonary hypertension
1974	Jejuno-ileal bypass	Liver failure
1978	Collagen-based VLCD	Deaths
1980	VLCD	Gallstones
1997	Fenfluramine/phentermine	Valvular insufficiency
2000	Phenylpropanolamine	Hemorrhagic stroke

Figure 9.1 Disappointments associated with many drugs used to treat obesity during the twentieth century. This dismal past makes the need for careful evaluation of future drugs all the more important. VLCD, very low calorie diet

1. It produces dose-related reduction in body weight

2. The maximum weight loss exceeds 20% of initial weight

3. It lowers blood pressure more than can be accounted for by weight loss

4. It lowers blood glucose more than can be accounted for by weight loss

5. It raises HDL-cholesterol and lowers triglycerides

6. It reduces visceral fat more than subcutaneous fat

7. It has only minimal side-effects

8. It produces no serious complications

9. It cannot be abused

10. It needs to be given only once daily

11. It does not interact with any other medication

12. It is inexpensive

Figure 9.2 Characteristics of an ideal drug

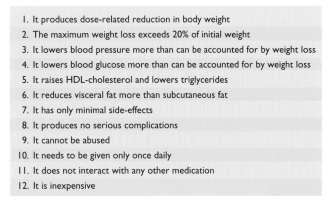

Figure 9.3 The first law of thermodynamics can be used to identify the places where drug treatment can work. Using this diagram, the mechanisms can be divided into those that affect food intake, those that affect energy expenditure and those that affect the metabolic interrelation between food intake and energy expenditure

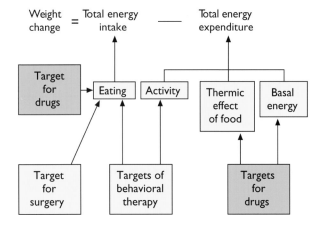

Monoamine	Mechanism	Examples
Noradrenergic	α-1 Agonist	Phenylpropanolamine
	α-2 Antagonist	Yohimbine
	β-2 Agonist	Clenbuterol
	Stimulate NE release	Phentermine
	Block NE reuptake	Mazindol
Serotonergic	5-HT 1B or 1C agonist	Quipazine
	Stimulate 5-HT release	Fenfluramine
	Block reuptake	Fluoxetine
Dopaminergic	D-2 Agonist	Apomorphine
Histaminergic	H-1 Antagonist	Chlorpheniramine

Figure 9.4 Both the noradrenergic and serotonergic receptor systems have been the basis for drugs to treat obesity. They can work by releasing the endogenous neurotransmitter, by blocking its reuptake or as a direct agonist. NE, norepinephrine

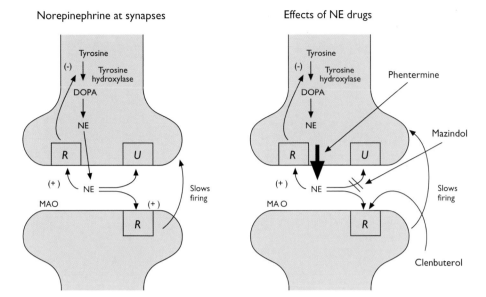

Figure 9.5 A noradrenergic nerve synapse. The norepinephrine (NE) in the storage granules is synthesized from tyrosine in a sequence where tyrosine hydroxylase is the rate-limiting enzyme. Once formed, the NE is stored in granules along with ATP until released into the neuronal cleft when the nerve ending is 'activated'. The NE that is released will diffuse to the receptors (R) and activate the adjacent nerve terminal. The NE can then be taken back up into the endplate (U) and deaminated or it can be methylated by catechol-O-methyl transferase (COMT). Drugs can act on this process by stimulating NE release, by blocking NE reuptake, by modulating monoamine oxidase (MAO) that deaminates the NE or by modulating the activity of COMT

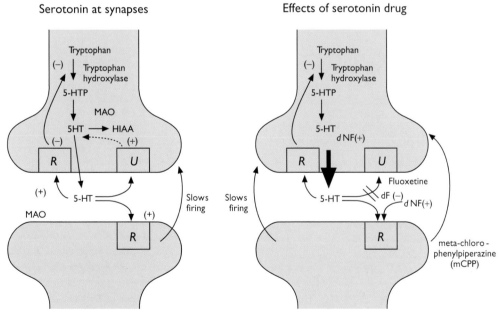

Figure 9.6 A serotonergic nerve synapse. The serotonin (5-hydroxytryptamine, 5-HT) in the storage granules is synthesized from tryptophan in the nerve terminal, but the rate-limiting step is the transport of tryptophan across the blood–brain barrier. Once formed, the 5-HT is stored in granules along with ATP until released into the neuronal cleft when the nerve ending is 'activated'. The 5-HT that is released will diffuse to the receptors (R) and activate the adjacent nerve terminal. The 5-HT can then be taken back up into the endplate (U). Drugs can act on this process by stimulating 5-HT release, by blocking 5-HT reuptake or by modulating monoamine oxidase (MAO) that deaminates the 5-HT. dF, d-fenfluramine; dNF, d-norfenfluramine

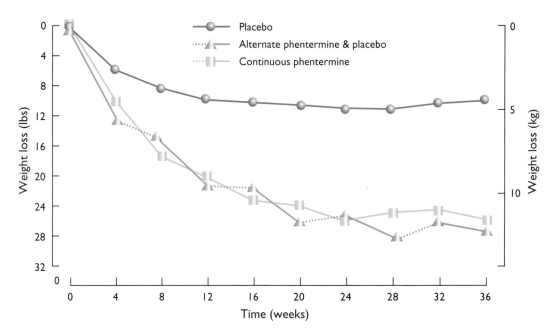

Figure 9.7 Weight loss with a noradrenergic drug. This 36-week, randomized, controlled clinical trial compared phentermine given daily, phentermine given daily on alternating months and placebo. Both groups treated with phentermine lost more weight than those receiving placebo, but there was no advantage of continuous over intermittent therapy. Note that about two-thirds of the weight loss was produced in the first 12 weeks and that no more weight loss was seen after 24 weeks. This plateau reflects the response of counter-regulatory mechanisms to preserve body mass. This drug has now been withdrawn from the market in Europe and is restricted to use for 'a few weeks' in the United States. Adapted with permission from Munro JF, MacCuish AC, Wilson EM, *et al*. Comparison of continuous and intermittent anorectic therapy in obesity. *Br Med J* 1968;1:352–4

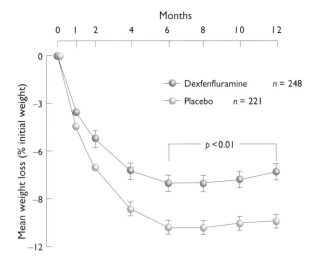

Figure 9.8 Serotonergic drugs also produce weight loss. Fenfluramine and dexfenfluramine are drugs that enhance serotonin release and block its reuptake. The first major multicenter trial, the International Dexfenfluramine (INDEX) trial, a drug that is no longer available due to cardiovascular side-effects, is shown here. The placebo-treated group lost about 7% of their body weight and the dexfenfluramine-treated patients about 10%. The plateau after 6 months of treatment is again evident. Adapted with permission of Elsevier Science from Guy-Grand B, Apfelbaum M, Crepaldi G, *et al*. International trial of long-term dexfenfluramine in obesity. *Lancet* 1989;2:1142–4

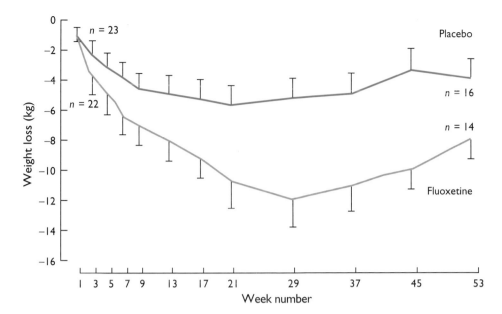

Figure 9.9 Drugs that block selectively serotonin reuptake are a second class of serotonergic drugs that have been tried in obesity. Data from a 52-week clinical trial of fluoxetine versus placebo are presented in this figure. Patients treated with fluoxetine lost weight during the first 20 weeks, but then regained weight over the next 32 weeks to a level not significantly different from control. This drug has not been approved by regulatory agencies for use in obesity. Adapted with permission from Darga LL, Carroll-Michals L, Botsford SJ, Lucas CP. Fluoxetine's effect on weight loss in obese subjects. *Int J Obes* 1992;16:193–8

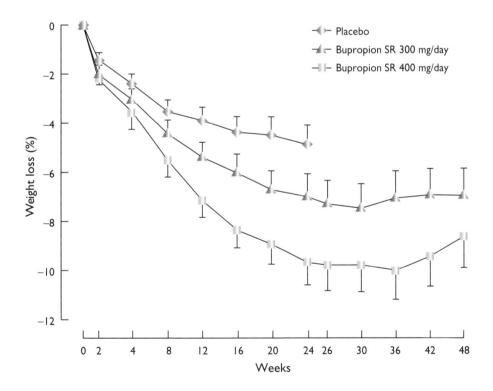

Figure 9.10 An antidepressant that reduces body weight. Bupropion is an approved antidepressant that was noted to reduce food intake. A double-blind clinical trial showed that it produced significantly greater weight loss than placebo. SR, sustained release. Adapted with permission from Anderson JW, Greenway FL, Fujioka K, *et al.* Bupropion SR enhances weight loss: a 48-week double-blind, placebo-controlled trial. *Obes Res* 2002;10:633–41

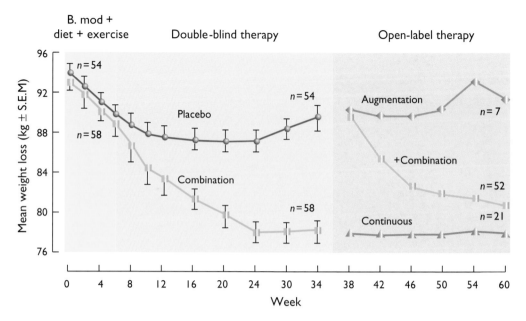

Figure 9.11 Since both noradrenergic and serotonergic drugs produce weight loss it was only a matter of time before the two types of drugs were combined. The first 52 weeks from a 3.5 year controlled clinical trial comparing the combination of phentermine, a noradrenergic drug, and fenfluramine, a sero-tonergic drug, is shown here. The weight loss in the placebo-treated patients at 32 weeks was 4.9% below baseline compared to 14.9% for those treated with the combination of drugs. When the placebo-treated patients were given the combination drugs during the next 6 months their weight loss reached that of the group initially treated with drugs. Adapted from Weintraub M. Long term weight control. The National Heart, Lung and Blood Institute funded multimodal intervention study. *Clin Pharmacol Ther* 1992;51:581–5, © 1992 with permission of Elsevier Science

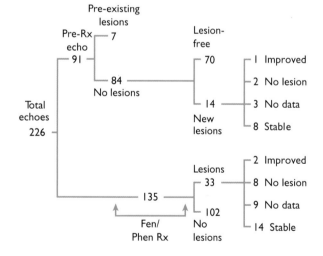

Figure 9.12 This combination of drugs met with the 'law of unintended consequences'. A significant number of patients receiving phentermine (Phen) and fenfluramine (Fen) for more than 6 months developed aortic valvulopathy with regurgitation. In this prospective study 25% of treated patients had aortic regurgitation with 16% of them developing it during treatment and some showing reversal after the drug was discontinued. Based on this problem fenfluramine was withdrawn from the worldwide market in 1997. Data derived from Ryan DH, Bray GA, Helmcke F, *et al.* Serial echocardiographic and clinical evaluation of valvular regurgitation before, during and after treatment with fenfluramine or dexfenfluramine and mazindol or phentermine. *Obes Res* 1999;7:313–22

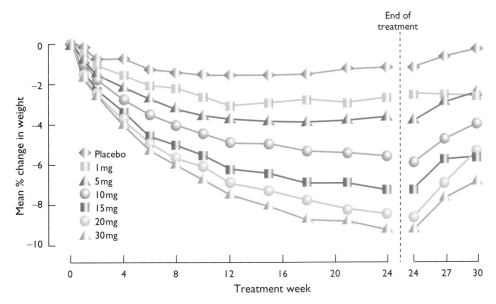

Figure 9.13 In the wake of this problem a new group of drugs have been developed and tested. The first was sibutramine. A 24-week, multi-dose, randomized, controlled clinical trial of sibutramine is shown here. There was a clear graded dose-response to sibutramine. When the drug was discontinued there was weight regain, indicating that the weight reduction at 24 weeks was a reflection of continuing drug effect, and that weight regain represented the loss of this effect. Adapted with permission from Bray GA, Blackburn GL, Ferguson JM, *et al.* Sibutramine produces dose-related weight loss. *Obes Res* 1999;7:189–98

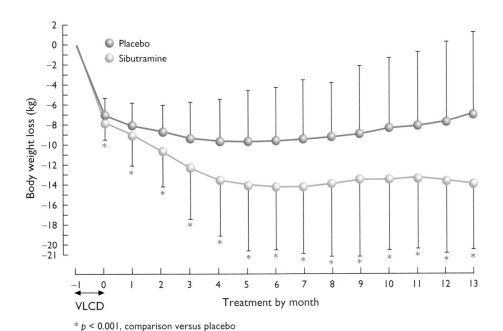

* *p* < 0.001, comparison versus placebo

Figure 9.14 The second trial of sibutramine. A 52-week, randomized, controlled clinical trial of sibutramine. Following an initial weight loss with a very low calorie diet (VLCD), patients were randomized to either placebo or 10 mg/day of sibutramine for 52 weeks. The drug-treated patients lost nearly 14% of their weight from baseline at 52 weeks, compared to a small regain in the placebo-treated patients. Adapted from Apfelbaum M, Vague P, Ziegler O, *et al.* Long-term maintenance of weight loss after a very-low-calorie diet: a randomized blinded trial of the efficacy and tolerability of sibutramine. *Am J Med* 1999;106:179–84, ©1999 with permission of Excerpta Medica Inc.

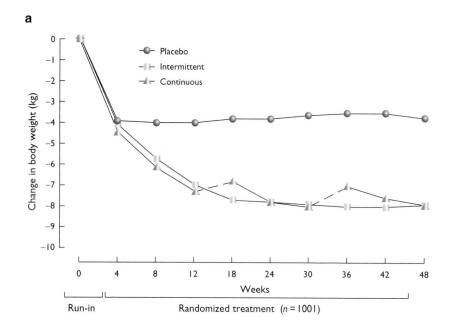

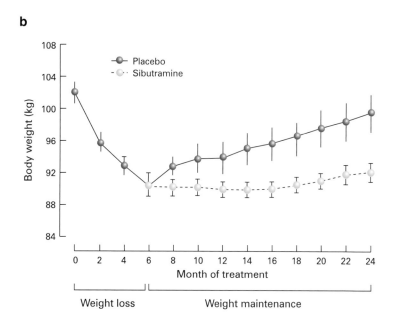

Figure 9.15 (a) Effect of intermittent and continuous therapy with sibutramine. Simiar to what was seen for phentermine in Figure 9.7, this 1-year trial of sibutramine 15 mg given continuously or intermittently with two 6-week hiatuses (weeks 12–18 and 30–36) produced the same overall weight loss as the drug given continuously. Data taken from Wirth A, Krause J. Long-term weight loss with sibutramine: a randomized clinical trial. *J Am Med Assoc* 2001;286:1331–9. (b) Two-year controlled clinical trial of sibutramine. All patients were treated with sibutramine 10 mg/day for the first 6 months in an open-label fashion. Those who lost more than 5 kg were then randomized into placebo- or sibutramine-treated groups for the next 18 months. Weight regain was steady in the placebo-treated patients, whereas the sibutramine-treated patients maintained most of their weight loss. Adapted with permission of Elsevier Science from James WPT, Astrup A, Finer N, *et al.*, for the STORM study group. Effect of sibutramine on weight maintenance after weight loss: a randomized trial. *Lancet* 2000;356: 2119–25

Side-effect	Noradrenergic	Serotonergic
Dry mouth	Yes	Yes
Decreased appetite	Yes	Yes
Constipation	Yes	No
Insomnia	Yes	Yes
Diarrhea	No	Yes
Palpitations	Yes	No
Increase in blood poessure	Yes	No

Figure 9.16 Side-effects of noradrenergic and serotonergic drugs

Clinical trial	Duration (months)	Drug or diet		Placebo or control	
		Δwt (%)	ΔDBP (mm Hg)	Δwt (%)	ΔDBP (mm Hg)
Hypertensive patients					
Sibutramine (Ca channel blockers)	12	−4.7	+2.0	−0.7	−1.3
Sibutramine (ACE inhibitors)	12	−4.8	+3.0	−0.3	−0.1
Sibutramine (β–blockers)	3	−4.5	+1.7	−0.4	+1.3
HPT	12	−4.7	−4.3	+0.4	−3.1
TOHP	12	−3.6	−5.8	+0.4	−3.8
Normotensive patients					
Sibutramine	6	−5.8	+3.4	−0.9	+1.7
Sibutramine	6	−8.7	+0.8	−4.2	−1.1
Orlistat	12	−10.2	−2.1	−6.1	+0.2
Orlistat	12	−9.7	−0.9	−6.6	−1.3
Orlistat	12	−8.8	−1.0	−5.8	+1.3
Orlistat	12	−7.9	−1.0	−4.2	+2.0

Figure 9.17 Effect of sibutramine on blood pressure. One of the most important side-effects of sibutramine is an increase in bood pressure which can lead to its discotinuance in a small number of patients. Four trials of sibutramine in hypertensive patients have been reported. This figure compares the weight loss and change in blood pressure of the placebo- and sibutramine-treated groups. As a comparison there are data from normotensive patients treated with sibutramine, obese patients treated with orlistat and hypertensive patients treated with diet. The patients treated with sibutramine had a small reduction of blood pressure or an increase of blood pressure relative to the other groups. HPT, Hypertension Prevention Trial; TOHP, Trials of Hypertension Prevention. Adapted with permission from Bray GA. Sibutramine and blood pressure: a therapeutic dilemma. *J Hum Hypertens* 2002;16:1–3

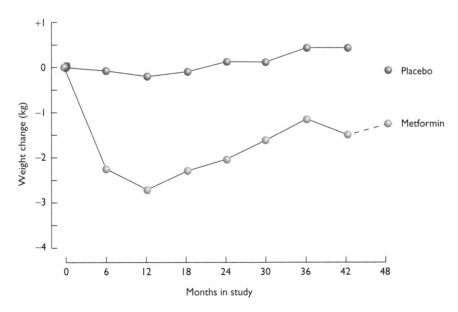

Figure 9.18 Effect of metformin on weight loss. Metformin is widely used in the treatment of diabetics. In contrast to sulfonylurea drugs and insulin, metformin actually produces weight loss. This double-blind, randomized trial compares metformin and placebo in patients with impaired glucose tolerance (IGT). There was a 31% reduction in the conversion rate from IGT to diabetes in those treated with metformin. Adapted with permission from Knowler WC, Barrett-Connor E, Fowler SE, *et al.* Reduction in the incidence of type 2 diabetes with lifestyle intervention or metformin. *N Engl J Med* 2002;346:393–403, © 2002 Massachusetts Medical Society. All rights reserved

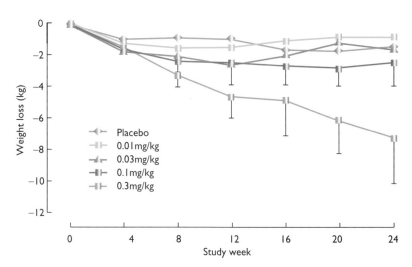

Figure 9.19 Leptin has been tried in the treatment of obesity. This figures shows a dose-ranging study where the highest dose showed modest, but significant, weight loss. Adapted with permission from Heymsfield SB, Greenberg AS, Fujioka K, *et al.* Recombinant leptin for weight loss in obese and lean adults: a randomized, controlled, dose-escalation trial. *J Am Med Assoc* 1999;282:1568–75

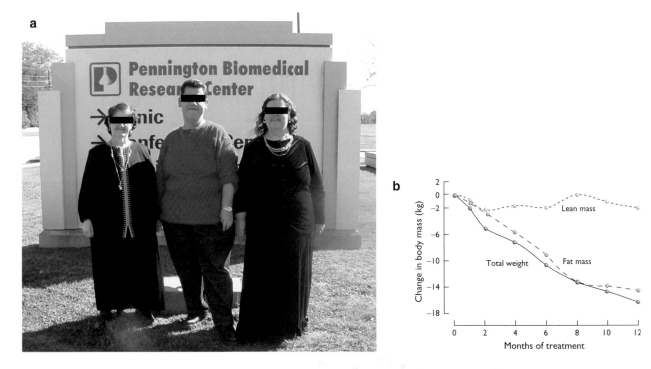

Figure 9.20 (a) Three cousins who are the only adults in the world known to be leptin-deficient. These individuals provided ideal subjects for researchers to study the effect of leptin in the absence of any existing endogenous leptin. All three cousins demonstrated voracious appetites prior to receiving medical help. Following treatment with leptin injections administered over a period of 10 months, all three subjects experienced considerable weight loss. Courtesy of Dr. Eric Ravussin. (b) Several leptin-deficient subjects show sustained responses to treatment with leptin, losing large amounts of weight. Leptin has not been approved for clinical use. Adapted with permission from Farooqi IS, Jebb SA, Langmack G, *et al.* Effects of recombinant leptin therapy in a child with congenital leptin deficiency. *N Engl J Med* 1999;341:879–84, ©1999 Massachusetts Medical Society. All rights reserved

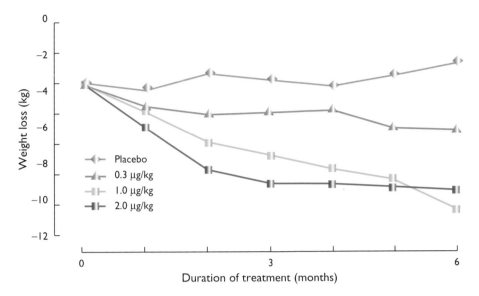

Figure 9.21 Ciliary neurotrophic factor is a second peptide that was studied in a clinical trial. In this short 12 week trial there was a dose-related decrease in body weight. This drug has not been approved for treating obesity. Data derived from Guler HP, Ettinger MP, Littlejohm TW, *et al.* Axokine causes significant weight loss in severely and morbidly obese subjects. *Int J Obes Relat Metab Disord Int* 2001;25(Suppl.1)S111(abstr.)

Glucagon-like peptide-1
• Decreases food intake in animals and man, peripherally and centrally
• Dose-dependent effect (−750 ± 200 kJ)
• Decreases gastric emptying
• Similar response in obese and lean

Figure 9.22 Glucagon-like peptide-1 which is formed by the gut during processing of proglucagon reduces food intake when given by intravenous infusion to human subjects. A number of clinical trials have recently been summarized and are presented in this table. No drugs in this class are approved for use in treating obesity. Data derived from Verdich C, Flint A, Gutzwiller JP, *et al.* A meta-analysis of the effect of glucagon-like peptide-1 (7–36) amide on ad libitum energy intake in humans. *J Clin Endocrinol Metab* 2001;86:4382–9

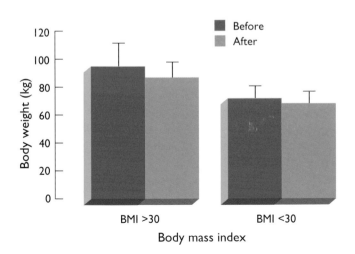

Figure 9.23 Results of a randomized, placebo-controlled, 6-month, dose-ranging clinical trial with topiramate, an anti-epileptic drug. Doses were increased stepwise, so that the highest dose reached its plateau by 12 weeks and was continued for an additional 12 weeks. Data derived from Bray G, Klein S, Levy B, *et al.* Topiramate produces dose-related weight loss in obese patients. *Diabetes* 2002;51(Suppl.1):A420–1

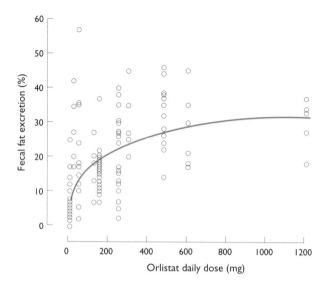

Figure 9.24   The only drug in the class of lipase inhibitors is orlistat which has been approved for marketing in most countries. It blocks pancreatic lipase in the intestine. Orlistat affects fecal fat loss. Subjects eating a 30 g fat diet were given increasing doses of orlistat and fecal fat loss was measured. At doses above 400 mg/day the fecal fat loss plateaued at about 30% of the dietary fat intake. Data derived from Zhi J, Melia AT, Guerciolini R, *et al.* Retrospective population-based analysis of the dose–response (fecal fat excretion) relationship of orlistat in normal and obese volunteers. *Clin Pharmacol Ther* 1994; 56:82–5

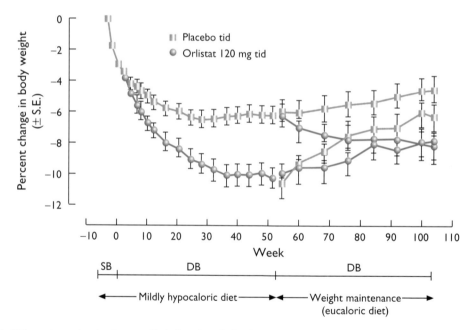

Figure 9.25   A 104-week, randomized, controlled clinical trial of orlistat. During the first year, patients received placebo, 60 mg not shown here or 120 mg of orlistat three times daily with meals, along with a diet with 30% fat that was reduced in energy by 500 kcal/day below maintenance. During the second year, patients were rerandomized to orlistat or placebo. Patients who remained on placebo throughout had the same weight as those who were switched from orlistat to placebo after 1 year. Similarly those on orlistat for 2 years had the same final weight as patients on orlistat only after the second year. SB, single-blind, DB, double-blind. Adapted with permission of Elsevier Science from Sjostrom L, Rissanen A, Andersen T, *et al.* Randomised placebo controlled trial of orlistat for weight loss and prevention of weight regain in obese patients. European Multicentre Orlistat Study Group. *Lancet* 1998;352:167–72

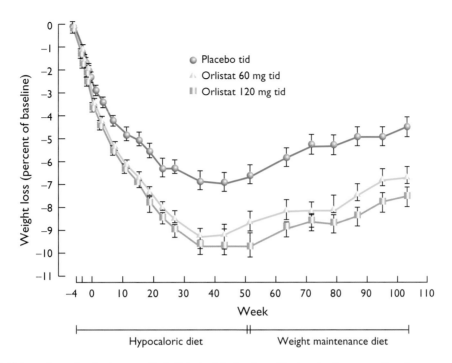

Figure 9.26 A 104-week, randomized, controlled clinical trial of orlistat. During the first year all patients were given a weight loss diet targeted for a reduction of 500 kcal/day below the maintenance energy level. During the second year all patients were assigned to a weight maintenance diet. During both years patients remained in either the placebo-treated of orlistat-treated groups receiving 60 or 120 mg three times a day with meals. Adapted with permission from Rossner S, Sjostrom L, Noack R, *et al.*, on behalf of the European Orlistat Obesity Study Group. Weight loss, weight maintenance, and improved cardiovascular risk factors after 2 years treatment with orlistat for obesity. *Obes Res* 2000;8:49–61

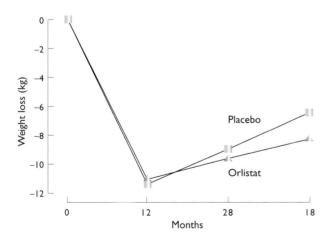

Figure 9.27 A 52-week, randomized, controlled trial of orlistat. Patients who lost at least 5 kg were randomized to receive either placebo, 30, 60 or 120 mg of orlistat three times daily with a 30% fat diet. The weight regain was significantly less in the patients treated with the highest dose of orlistat compared to placebo, as shown here, but not with the two lower doses. Data derived from Hill JO, Hauptmann J, Anderson JW, *et al.* Orlistat, a lipase inhibitor, for weight mainternance after conventional dieting: a 1 year study. *Am J Clin Nutr* 1999;69: 1108–16

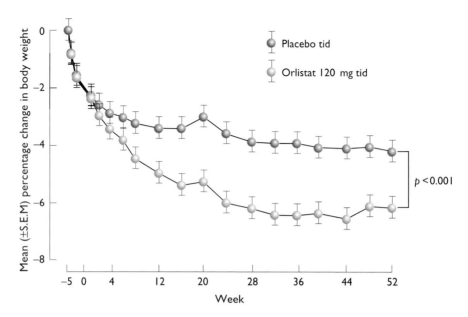

Figure 9.28 Effect of orlistat for 1 year on weight loss in diabetic patients whose diabetes was controlled primarily with sulfonyl-ureas. The placebo- and drug-treated patients both received a calorie-reduced diet with 30% of calories from fat. Orlistat was given in a dose of 120 mg in three divided doses. The drug-treated patients lost significantly more weight than the placebo-treated patients. Adapted with permission of The American Diabetes Association from Hollander P, Elbein SC, Hirsch IB, *et al.* Role of orlistat in the treatment of obese patients with type 2 diabetes. A 1-year randomized double-blind study. *Diabetes Care* 1998;21:1288–94, ©1998 American Diabetes Association

	Year 1 (%)			Year 2 (%)		
	Placebo	Orlistat	Withdrawal	Placebo	Orlistat	Withdrawal
Oily spotting	1	27	1.7	0.2	4	0.2
Flatus & discharge	1	24	0.6	0.2	2	0.2
Fecal urgency	7	22	0.3	2.0	3	0.0
Fatty/oily stool	3	20	0.1	1.0	6	0.3
Oily evacuation	1	12	0.0	0.2	2	0.0
Increased defecation	4	11	0.3	1.0	3	0.0
Fecal incontinence	1	8	1.1	0.2	2	0.2

Figure 9.29 As a drug that blocks pancreatic lipase, the side-effects of orlistat are predictable. They include a variety of gastro-intestinal complaints that only occasionally lead to discontinuation of the drug. These complications are seen most frequently in the first 3 months of therapy

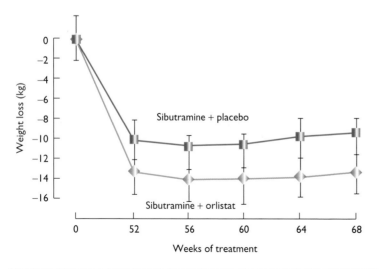

Figure 9.30 The development of sibutramine and orlistat that work by different mechanisms suggested that they might be additive. When orlistat and placebo were added to patients who had received sibutramine for 12 months, there was no further weight loss and no effect of the added orlistat. Adapted with permission from Wadden TA, Berkowitz RK, Womble LG, *et al.* Effects of sibutramine plus orlistat in obese women following 1 year of treatment by sibutramine alone: a placebo-controlled trial. *Obes Res* 2000;8:431–7

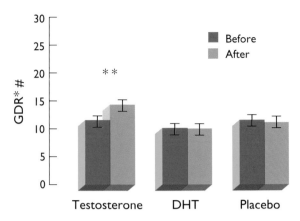

*GDR: Glucose disappearance rate during glucose
clamp (mg × kg LBM^{-1} × min^{-1})
**$p < 0.01$ (ANOVA, before–after treatment)
#Differences between treatment effects within groups
measured with Kruskal–Wallis' non-parametric test, $p < 0.05$

Figure 9.31 Both growth hormone and testosterone decrease visceral fat. The changes observed with testosterone in men with lower levels of testosterone are shown here. This use of testosterone has not been approved. Data derived from Marin P, Holmang S, Gustafsson C, *et al.* Androgen treatment of abdominally obese men. *Obes Res* 1993;1:245–51

Figure 9.32 Increasing the expenditure of energy by increasing the metabolism is another mechanism for drugs to treat obesity. This figure shows a 6-month, randomized, placebo-controlled trial in 180 patients treated with ephedrine 20 mg three times daily, caffeine 200 mg three times daily, a placebo or the combination of ephedrine and caffeine. During the first 6 months when the study was double-blind, the patients treated with ephedrine and caffeine lost significantly more weight than those in the other three groups. During the 6-month, open-lable extension when all patients received the combination of ephedrine and caffeine they all reached a similar weight. Adapted with permission from Astrup A, Breum L, Toubro S, *et al.* The effect and satiety of an ephedrine/caffeine compound compared to ephedrine, caffeine and placebo in obese subjects on an energy restricted diet. A double-blind trial. *Int J Obes* 1992;16:269–77

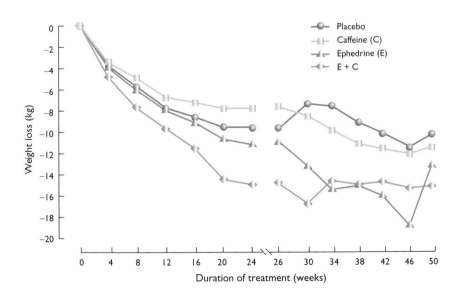

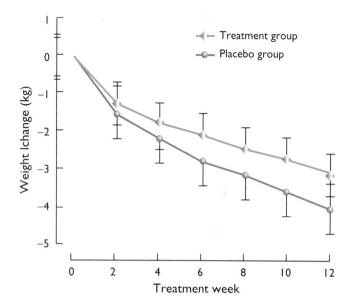

Figure 9.33 Hydroxycitrate, a chemical that blocks citrate lyase, was shown to produce weight loss in animals. In human beings, a herbal product from *Garcinia cambogia* which provides hydroxycitrate was compared to placebo. There was no difference in the amount of weight loss observed. Adapted from Heymsfield SB, Allison DB, Vasselli JR, *et al. Garcinia cambofia* (hydroxycitric acid) as a potential antiobesity agent: a randomized controlled trial. *J Am Med Assoc* 1998;280:1596–600, ©1998 American Medical Association

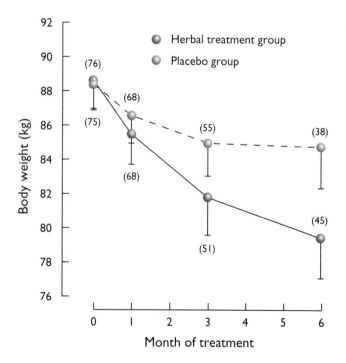

Figure 9.34 Herbal products that supply thermogenic products similar to ephedrine and caffeine have been tested in two clinical trials. During the 6 months of treatment, the product containing ephedra from Ma huang and caffeine from Kola nut produced more weight loss than the control. Adapted with permission from Boozer CN, Daly PA, Homel P, *et al.* Herbal ephedra/caffeine for weight loss: a 6-month randomized safety and efficacy trial. *Int J Obes* 2002;26:593–604

Drug group	FDA approval	Approved duration of treatment	DEA schedule	Trade names	Dosage form (mg)	Administration
Sympathomimetic drugs approved for short-term use (schedule IV)						
Diethylpropion (United States)	Yes	Few weeks	IV	Tenuate® Tenuate® Dospan®	25 75	25 mg three times daily 75 mg once daily
Phentermine (United States)	Yes	Few weeks	IV	Standard Adipex-P® Duromine Fastin® Obenix® Oby-Cap® Oby-Trim Zantryl Slow release Ionamin®	37.5 30 37.5 30 30 30 15, 30	37.5 mg/in am 30 mg/day 2h after breakfast 37.5mg/day 9am 30 mg/day 2h after breakfast 30 mg/day 2h after breakfast 30 mg/day 2h after breakfast 15 mg/day before breakfast (30 mg for less responsive patients)
Sympathomimetic drugs approved for long-term use *Serotonin–norepinephrine reuptake inhibitor*						
Sibutramine	Yes	Long-term	IV	Meridia Reductil	5, 10, 15	Initial dose, 10 mg/day maximum dose 15 mg/day
Pancreatic lipase inhibitor approved for long-term use						
Orlistat	Yes	Long-term	n/a	Xenical	120	120 mg three times a day with meals

Figure 9.35 Table of medications available in the United States. This will vary from country to country depending on regulatory agencies. There are several drugs that are only approved for a few weeks in the United States and that may not be available in other countries. The two drugs approved for long-term use are approved in most countries. The decision to use medications depends on whether the patient has 'clinical overweight'. This means a BMI > 30 or BMI > 27 with such problems as hypertension, diabetes, low HDL-cholesterol and high triglycerides, increased central fat or sleep apnea. During the induction of initial weight with the primary treatments, medications can be added if the patient is in medical need. Data derived from Bray GA. Drug treatment of obesity. *Rev Endocr Metab Disord* 2001;2:403–18 and Yanovski SZ, Yanovski JA. Obesity. *N Engl J Med* 2002;346:591–602

WARNING: Most drugs for the treatment of obesity are scheduled by the US Drug Enforcement Agency. Theses schedules and the FDA guidelines are used by state regulatory agencies to develop regulations for medical practice which have the force of law. Use of any scheduled drug in a manner different from these regulations, regardless of whether it is reasonable medical practice or in the patient's best interest can result in criminal prosecution for a felony offense. Whether or not the regulations are based on truth, you can go to jail or have your license suspended. If you intend to use these drugs check the regulations in force in your state!

Figure 9.36 Drug treatment of obesity: warning

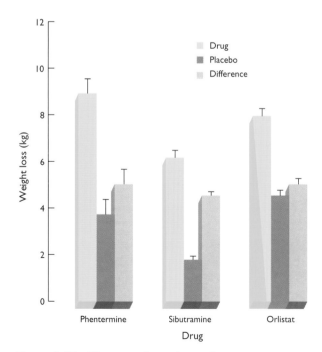

Figure 9.37 Effect size of anti-obesity drugs

Operations for obesity in humans	
1954	Jejunoileal small bowel bypass
1963	Jejunocolic bypass
1967	Gastric bypass
1971	Gastroplasty
1978	Gastric banding or wrapping
1978	Truncal vagotomy
1979	Biliopancreatic bypass
1981	Vertical-banded gastroplasty
1981	Biliointestinal bypass
1982	Ileogastrostomy
1983	Intestinal interposition
1986	Esophageal banding
1986	Adjustable gastric banding
1990	Laparoscopic banding

Figure 10.1 Operations for obesity in human beings

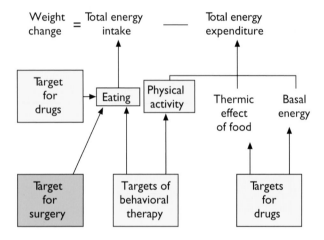

Figure 10.2 Energy balance diagram showing where surgical treatment has its influence

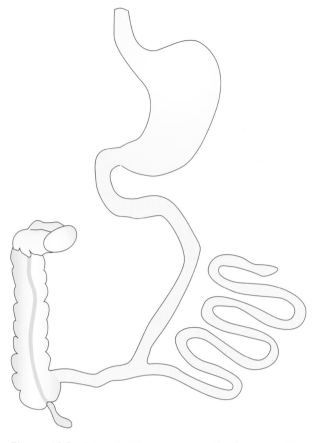

Figure 10.3 Jejunoileal bypasses were the first operations that were performed regularly for obesity. One was an end-side anastamosis (shown here) in which the proximal 25 cm of the cut end of the jejunum was attached to the side of the ileum about 10 cm from the ileocecal valve. The other operation was an end-to-end anastamosis with 35 cm of jejunum attached to the ileum end-to-end 10 cm from the ileocecal valve. The blind loop drained into the colon. The large blind loop produced by either operation was associated with a variety of metabolic symptoms of which hepatic failure was the most important. For these reasons the operation has been abandoned

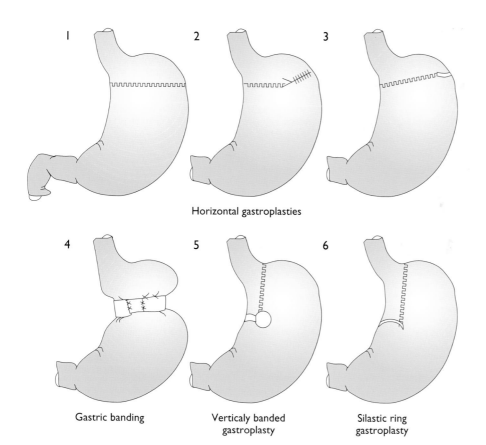

Horizontal gastroplasties

Gastric banding

Verticaly banded
gastroplasty

Silastic ring
gastroplasty

Figure 10.4 A diagram of the gastric restriction operations. Of these the vertically banded gastroplasty is the most popular (number 5). It is basically an extension of the esophagus into a small upper gastric pouch with a lower constriction. The vertically banded gastroplasty is relatively easy to perform with surgical stapling instruments, but the resulting weight loss is less than that with the gastric bypass operation described below. Adapted with permission of the American Journal of Clinical Nutrition from Grace DM. Gastric restriction procedures for treating severe obesity. *Am J Clin Nutr* 1992;55: 5565–95, © American Journal of Clinical Nutrition/American Society for Clinical Nutrition

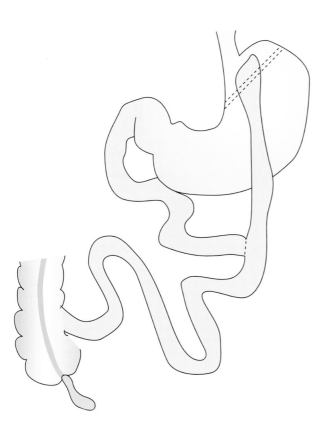

Figure 10.5 A diagram of the Roux-en-Y gastric bypass operation. In this procedure a loop of jejunum is attached to a small 50 ml upper gastric pouch and the duodenum is attached to this jejunal loop further down. The weight loss with this operation is superior to the vertically banded gastroplasty described above

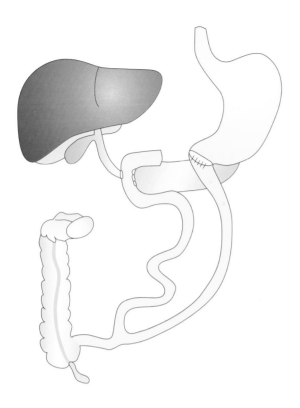

Figure 10.6 A diagram of the biliopancreatic operation often referred to as the Scopinaro procedure. In this procedure the stomach and the lower jejunum are transected. The duodenal-jejunal region is reattached to the ileum near the ileocecal valve. The other limb is attached to the small upper gastric pouch. With this procedure more malabsorption is produced. The degree of malabsorption can be controlled by varying the lengths of each intestinal segment and the points at which the flow is reattached in the ileum

Complication	Vertical gastroplasty	Roux-en-Y Gastric bypass	Biliopancreatic diversion
	% of patients		
Weight loss (% excess body weight at 3 year)	40–63%	68–72% (55 at 10 year)	75% (77 at 10 year)
Mortality (perioperative)	0–1.0	0–2.5	0.5–1.0
Leak/sepsis	0–1	0–2.5	0–0.3
Outlet stenosis	4–20	3.5–22	3–5
Peptic ulceration	1–8	2.2–11	2.8
Malnutrition			7
Anemia		30–39	5–35
Mineral/vitamin deficits:			
Iron		28–56	
Folate		1.8–14	
B_{12}	17	22–37	
Staple disruption	1.7–48	1.6–8	——
Surgical revision(s)	41–45	1–10	1.7–20

Figure 10.7 Operative complications are common. This table lists the more common problems following surgery. As laparoscopic procedures replace open surgical operations the rates for all of these complications can be expected to continue to fall

Surgical treatment improves
Sleep apnea
Fertility
Urinary incontinence
Osteoarthritis
Pseudotumor cerebri
Quality of life
Employment opportunities

Figure 10.8 Benefits from weight loss induced by surgery

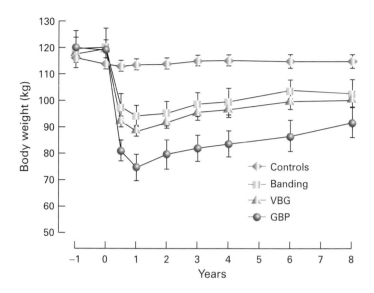

Figure 10.9 A comparison of weight loss with the gastric bypass (GBP), the vertically banded gastroplasty (VBG) and the silastic banded gastric restrictive operation. Shown are data on 232 obese controls and 251 surgically treated obese patients from matching until the end of year 8 in the Swedish Obese Subjects Study. The data are based on the patients who completed each time point. Adapted with permission from Sjostrom CD, Peltonen M, Wedel H, Sjostrom L. Differentiated long-term effects of intentional weight loss on diabetes and hypertension. Hypertension 2000;36:20-25

Parameter	Men (n = 214)			Women (n = 241)		
	Baseline	2 years	Δ	Baseline	2 years	Δ
Age (years)	47.2 ± 5.7	—	—	47.6 ± 6.0	—	—
Weight (kg)	129.7 ± 17	106.5 ± 19	−23.2	113.8 ± 14	93.5 ± 17	−26.3
BMI (kg/m²)	40.6 ± 47	33.3 ± 5.6	− 7.3	42.0 ± 4.0	34.5 ± 5.8	−7.5
SBP (mmHg)	144 ± 18	137 ± 19	− 7	144 ± 19	137 ± 19	−7
DBP (mmHg)	91 ± 11	85 ± 10	− 6	88 ± 11	83 ± 9.5	−5
TG (mmol/l)	2.87 ± 2.4	1.96 ± 1.6	−0.91	2.08 ± 1.2	1.67 ± 1.0	−0.41
Glu (mmol/l)	5.8 ± 2.3	4.9 ± 2.0	−0.9	5.5 ± 2.1	4.7 ± 1.7	−0.8
Ins(mmol/l)	25.9 ±14.8	13.7 ± 9.3	−12.2	20.7 ± 11.8	11.6 ± 7.7	−9.1
Uric (μmol/l)	419 ± 82	358 ± 90	− 61	356 ± 80	295 ± 76	−61
Chol (mmol/l)	6.1 ± 1.2	5.6 ± 1.2	− 0.5	5.9 ± 1.1	5.8 ± 1.1	−0.1
HDL (mmol/l)	1.06 ± 0.23	1.18 ± 0.30	+ 0.12	1.23 ± 0.29	1.35 ± 0.32	+0.12

Figure 10.10 Surgical weight reduction reduces the incident cases of diabetes, hypertension and insulin resistance during the first 2 years. After a follow-up of 4 or more years the reduction in new cases of diabetes is very striking, but blood pressure returns to control levels. BMI, body mass index: SBP, systolic blood pressure; DBP, diastolic blood pressure; TG, triglycerides; Glu, glucose; Ins, insulin; Uric, uric acid; Chol, cholesterol; HDL, high-density lipoprotein

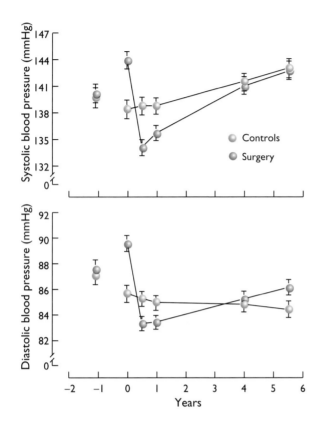

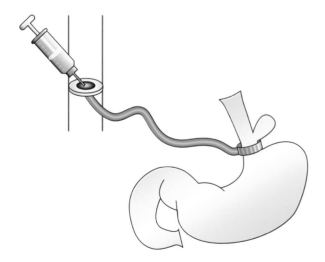

Figure 10.11 The pattern of change in blood pressure over the first 6 years of the Swedish Obese Subjects study is shown. There was an initial decrease that had returned to baseline by 4–6 years and remained there thereafter. Adapted with permission from Sjostrom CD, Peltonen M, Sjostrom L. Blood pressure during long-term weight loss in the obese: the Swedish Obese Subjects (SOS) Intervention Study. *Obes Res* 2001;9:188–95

Figure 10.12 This figure shows the laparoscopically placed gastric band that is commercially available. A comparison of weight loss with this procedure versus other procedures is shown in Figure 10.9

Index

A
α Receptors 18
ABC Scheme 90
abdomen, CT scans 43
absorptiometer, X-ray 42
adrenalectomy 20
aerobic activity and heart rate rise 106
afferent signals 17–18
agouti-related peptide 18, 52
Ahlstrom syndrome and obesity 80
American Cancer Society Study II 59
amphetamine 14, 21–2
amphetamines 23
anticonvulsants, and obesity 77
antidepressants
    for body weight reduction 24, 113
    and obesity 77
antidiabetic drugs, and obesity 77
aortic valvulopathy, after phentermine–
        fenfluramine combination 114
autonomic nervous system 20

B
ß2 Receptors 18
ß3-Adrenergic receptor 22
ß3-Adrenergic receptor agonists 16
ß-Adrenergic blockers, and obesity 77
Barbet–Biedl syndrome 80, 81
behavioral approaches to weight reduction 3, 90
behavioral predictors of weight loss 90
behavioral therapy
    and drug treatment, weight loss improvement 94
    in obesity treatment 90–1
    over internet 94
    structural eating plan 94
behavioral weight programs 91
    childhood 93
benzphetamine 23
biliopancreatic operation, diagram 128

blood pressure, pattern of change after
        surgery 130
Blount's disease, childhood 72
body
    fat and lean compartments and energy 44
    longitudinal CT scan 43
body composition
    levels 41
    measurement methods 43
    socioeconomic status 46
body fat
    age effects 44
    control, factor relationships 49
    distribution and age 45
    ethnicity, age and gender effects 46
body mass index
    cancer risk 69
    cardiovascular disease risk 65
    cholesterol
        and blood pressure relationship with
                mortality 67
        triglycerides higher levels 65
    and death risk increase 59
    determination from table 40
    ethnicity effects 46
    heart disease relationship 65
    higher, and diabetes risk 62
    inactivity relationship to 105
    increasing, gall bladder disease risk 69
    obesity classification by 41
    osteoarthritis development 71
body weight
    higher, and death risk increase 59
    and physical activity 16
bombesin 17
breast cancer model 69
breast feeding 26
    and overweight children 100
bupropion 24, 113

C

caffeine 23, 24
  side-effects 25
caffeine trial 123
calcium intake 26
calcium intake and body weight 101
calories
  counters 99
  deficit and weight loss 98
  intake analysis 97
  values in food 104
Cambridge Diet 22
carbohydrate oxidation 16
cardiac stress test 106
Carpenter syndrome and obesity 80
cholecystokinin 17, 52
ciliary neurotrophic factor 18
  clinical trial 119
citrate:ATP lyase 17
cocaine–amphetamine-regulated
    transcript 18, 52
Cohen syndrome and obesity 80
combination therapy 22
Committee on Proprietary Medicinal Products 13
cortisol 20
Craig, Jenny 22
Cushing's syndrome and obesity 76

D

dexfenfluramine 14, 18, 23–4, 112
diabetes, surgical weight reduction and case
    reduction 129
diabetes mellitus, non-insulin-dependent,
    childhood 72
diaglycerol transferase 17
diagnostic exercise tests 106
diet
  balanced deficit and low calorie 98
  books 99
  classification, and energy levels 96
  and energy balance 96
  low-fat 100
  recommended intake of nutrients 103
diet plan, physician's 92, 97
diethylpropion 23, 125
dinitrophenol 16, 21
dopamine receptors 19
drug
  anti-obesity, effect size 125
  ideal
    anti-obesity 25–7
    characteristics 110
    cost 26
    mechanism of action 26
    safety 25–6
dyslipidemias, childhood 72

E

eating behavior 91–2
  control and planning 95
efferent signals 19–20
endocrine disturbance and obesity 74
energy balance 15–17, 90, 96
  diagram 126
  and physical activity 104
energy expenditure 15
  by increasing metabolism 123
  with daily activities 108
  and fat-free body mass 55
  individual women 56
  measurement by double-labeled water 55
  and physical activity 104
  to maintain weight loss 109
energy intake, portion control 99
energy needs, estimation 97
enterostatin 17, 52
enzymes, in fat metabolism 17
ephedrine 23, 24
  side-effects 25
  trial 123
ephedrine/caffeine trial 123
epiphysis, slipped capital femoral, childhood 72
estrogens 19
ethnicity and disease risks 61
exercise
  increase 16
  to prevent weight regain 107
  and weight loss 106

F

fat
  brown, uncoupling protein (UCP1) 16
  central increase, mortality risk 60
  dietary, in obesity development 54
fat cells 57
  differentiation 16, 74
  as endocrine cell 62
  enlargement 73
  number of 74
  white, development 58
fat counting 99
fat stores and obesity 16
fatty acid secretion and diabetes 64
fatty acids, see also free fatty acids
fenfluramine 18, 22–3, 24, 112
FLUORIDE hypothesis 26–7
fluoxetine 22, 24, 113
food
  energy in 104
  for four for one year 55
  thermic effect, measurement 56
food groups and calories 102
food guide pyramid 101

food intake
  changes with age 53
  decrease and weight loss 20
  inhibition 52
  reduction, drugs for 23–4
  regulation 18
  sympathetic nervous system relationship 52
  stimulation 52
  timing mechanism 53
  variability 53
Framingham Study 71
free fatty acids
  see also fatty acids
  increased, risk factors 66
fructose 27
  high, corn sweeteners 54, 101

G
galanin 19
gall bladder disease, development, cholesterol
    metabolism model 70
gastric restriction operations 127
gastrin-releasing peptide 17
gastrointestinal peptides 17
genes, single, animal models 50
genetic factors, in obesity development 49
ghrelin 17, 51–2
glucagon 17
glucagon-like peptide-1 17, 52, 119
glucocorticoids 19–20
glucose
  level dip 18
    as timing mechanism 53
glycemic index 100
growth hormone 19–20, 24
  weight loss 123

H
herbal products, clinical trials 124
histamine receptors 19
3-hydroxybutyrate 17
hydroxycitrate 17, 124
hypertension
  childhood 72
  model, risk of development 68
  surgical weight reduction and case
      reduction 129
hypothalamus, lesions and obesity 74

I
insulin 16, 19–20
  and weight gain 78
insulin resistance
  in metabolic syndrome 64, 85
  surgical weight reduction and case reduction 129
  syndromes 64

International Dexfenfluramine (INDEX) trial 112
internet, behavioral therapy 94
intracranial pressure and obesity 74

J
janus kinase/signal translation and transduction
    pathway 18
jejunoileal bypasses 126

L
lactate 17
Lambert, Daniel 39
laparoscopy, gastric band 130
Last Chance Diet 22
leprechaunism 64
leptin 17–18, 23, 52
  clinical trials 118
  deficiency, cousins 118
  and obesity 57, 80, 118
  receptor deficiency, family tree 80
  role 58
lipoatrophy, total congenital 64
lipodystrophy, partial congenital 64

M
mazindol 14, 22, 23
medical examinations, guidelines 106
melanin concentrating hormone 51–2
  receptors 19
melanocortin receptor system 19
metabolism, drugs altering 24
metformin
  and weight gain 78
  weight loss effect 117
milk, low-fat, nutrition label 98
models, animal, single-gene defects 50
mouse
  diabetes 50
  fat 50
  obese 50, 79
  Tub 50
  yellow 50, 79

N
National Heart, Lung and Blood Institute
  clinical guidelines for treatment of obesity 41
  overweight evaluation algorithm 85
National Weight Control Registry 108
neuroleptics and obesity 77
neurological disturbances and obesity 74
neuromedin B 17
neuropeptide Y 18
neuropeptides 19
New England Journal of Medicine 22
noradrenergic drugs, side-effects 25, 116
noradrenergic nerve synapse 111

noradrenergic receptor systems, as drug
  basis 110, 112
norepinephrine 19, 52, 111
Nurses' Health Study 61

O
*Obesity: Preventing and Managing the Global
  Epidemic*, WHO 86
obesity
  anatomic characteristics 73
  associated risks 73
  cardiovascular disease risk 65
  central
    CT scan measurement 66
    and diabetes risk 63
    metabolic syndrome and insulin resistance 85
  childhood
    complications of obesity 72
    treatment strategies 88
  classification by BMI 41
  costs associated with 59
  development 51
    dietary fat role 54
    genetic factors 49
  disorders associated with 59
  drug treatment
    disappointments 110
    warning 125
  endocrine complications 70
  as epidemic 13–14
  etiologic classification 73
  etiology 15–20
  exercise treatment 107
  functional classification 73
  genetic factors 15
  hypothalamic, causes 74
  increasing prevalence, worldwide 48
  longevity effect 60
  and losing weight 72
  measurement methods 39
  progressive syndrome 83
  psychosocial difficulties 72
  surgical operations 126
    benefits 128
    complications 128
    disorder reduction 129
  human syndromes 79
  treatment 21–7
    drug side-effects 25
    drugs 23–5
    historical perspective 21–3
    mechanisms of action 23
    problems 14
    selection 13, 87
opioid receptors 19
Optifast program 22

orexin A 19
orlistat 17, 23, 24, 125
  1 year weight loss 122
  clinical trials 120–1
  daily dose 120
  effect size 125
  side-effects 25, 122

P
pancreatic peptides 17
patient
  obese
    health professional encounter 84
    identification from mortality ratios and life
      insurance data 84
    natural history 84
    pre-obese older, therapeutic strategies 89
peroxisome proliferator-activated receptor-γ 15
phendimetrazine 23
phenothiazines 19
phentermine 14, 22, 23, 35, 112
  effect size 125
phentermine/fenfluramine combination 114
  side-effects 114
phenylpropanolamine 18, 23
physical activity
  index 105
  pattern and longevity 105
*Physical Activity and Health: Report of the
  Surgeon General* 105
physical fitness and health risks 61
Planet Health Study 26
polycystic ovary syndrome
  childhood 72
  and obesity 77
Prader–Willi syndrome
  clinical findings 81
  and obesity 80
  treatment 88
pregnancy and weight gain 78
pro-opiomelanocortin 18, 52
  deficiency in childhood 82
pseudo-acromegaly 64
pyruvate 17

R
Rabson–Mendenhall syndrome 64
rat
  fatty 50, 79
  Koletsky 50
retinoid X receptor 16
Roux-en-Y gastric bypass operation 127

S
Scopinaro procedure 128
serotonergic drugs, side-effects 25, 116

serotonergic nerve synapse 111
serotonergic receptor systems, as drug
    basis 110, 112
serotonergic selective reuptake blocking drugs 113
serotonin system 18
sertraline 24
sibutramine 23–4, 125
    blood pressure effect 117
    effect size 125
    intermittent and continuous therapy effect 116
    trials 115
sibutramine/orlistat, development 122
sleep apnea 70
    childhood 72
smell receptors 17
soft drinks, consumption 26, 54
steroid hormones, and obesity 77
sugar sweetening and increased BMI in children 101
sulfonylureas and weight gain 78
Sweden, behavioral therapy study 93
Swedish Obese Subjects Study 63, 67
    blood pressure pattern of change 130
    surgical procedures 129
sympathetic nervous system 20, 52

taste receptors 17
television and overweight children 107–8
testosterone 19–20, 24
    weight loss 123
thermodynamics
    first law, and drug treatment mechanisms 110
    first law of 15
thermogenesis
    drugs increasing 24–5
    stimulation 16
thyroid extract 21
thyroid hormones 16, 19
topiramate, clinical trial 119
tuberculoma and obesity 75
tyrosine phosphatase-IB 16–17

U
UK Prospective Diabetes Study 78
uncoupling proteins 16, 56

urocortin 19
US
    obesity prevalence 47
        in adults 48
        in ethnic groups 48
US children, obesity prevalence 46
US Drug Enforcement Agency 14, 22
US Food and Drug Agency 23
US medications available 125
US National Center for Health Statistics 107
US soldiers, weight and height 46
uterine cancer model 69

V
venlafaxine 24
Venus of Willendorf 83

W
waist–hip ratio, central fat estimation 60
walking, to reduce weight 109
weighing compartment, underwater 42
weight gain
    and diabetes 62
    and increased mortality 61
    leptin-deficient children 80
    predictors 86
    therapy goals 87
    therapy selection algorithm 86
weight loss
    antidepressant for 113
    behavioral strategy intensity 93
    blood pressure reduction 68
    and calory reduction 97
    and diabetes metabolic variables 63
    and exercise 106
    and higher activity 108
    with meal replacements 99
    with noradrenergic drug 112
    programs, categories of success 87
    relationship to weight goals 89
    with serotonergic drugs 112
    surgical procedures 129
women, overweight, weight goals 72, 89
World Health Organization 1997,
        Consultation on Obesity 41